The L
Your

How to Improve with Age

The Life in Your Years

How to Improve with Age

SUSANNE O'LEARY

Newleaf

Newleaf

an imprint of
Gill & Macmillan Ltd
Hume Avenue, Park West, Dublin 12
with associated companies throughout the world
www.gillmacmillan.ie
© Susanne O'Leary 2000
0 7171 3082 7
Illustrations by Gemma Weir
Design and print origination by Design Image, Dublin
Printed in Malaysia

This book is typeset in 10/19pt Stone Sans

A CIP catalogue record for this book is available from the British Library.

1 3 5 4 2

To Denis

Contents

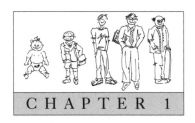

CHAPTER 1

INTRODUCTION
DON'T STOP!

Mae West is supposed to have said, 'It's not the men in my life that count, but the life in my men.' You could change that statement a little and apply it to life: *it's not the years in your life that count, but the life in your years.*

We all know we are going to die; but we don't know when (though certain health books give the impression that death is somehow optional). There is a trend in health literature to make us believe that by adopting a healthy life-style we can live to be a hundred. It is more realistic to claim that a healthy life-style slows down the ageing process and makes us feel well, thus improving the quality of life. It also helps us cope with hardships, and improves our ability to fight disease. A healthy life does not guarantee the absence of illness, but it can help make certain illnesses easier to cope with, and speed up recovery.

Many people fear old age; they often see it as the beginning of the end of life. Some people even seem to think that at a certain age they will have to give up things they enjoy and become a different person, someone who is 'old'. They often stop keeping physically active, and begin to watch the rest of the world from the outside; they no longer feel part of the world.

The word 'old' is in itself negative when applied to people. Old houses, antiques, cars and wine are things we admire, enjoy, and even desire; but we want old people to remove themselves from society and not to bother us (or remind us of the fact that we will ourselves be old one day). This is a great pity, because old people have much to offer, in wisdom, life experiences, and love. An old person can often be wonderful company. It's time that middle-aged and younger people made more of an effort to include old people in their circle of family and friends. Most people grow old, and will have to cope with negative attitudes themselves.

Life expectancy in the western world has risen by fifteen years since the nineteen-thirties; but the quality of life—that is to say, general health—has *not* improved. It may seem encouraging that many people now live to eighty and beyond; but what good are fifteen extra years if they are spent in long-term care? Why sit in an old people's home, ill and forgotten? If we look after our health, we can make sure the extra years are enjoyable and fulfilling. It is possible to keep active and alert into an advanced age. It is up to the individual to make it happen. It takes determination, hard work, and a certain amount of pain and discomfort.

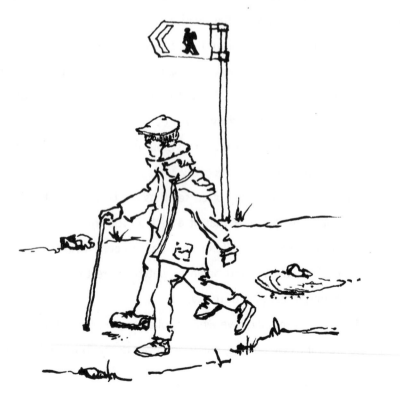

The three main components that are vital for a healthy life as you age are **attitude**, **effort**, and **nutrition**. You can improve your attitude to life, and in that way start making an effort to keep physically and mentally active. Learning about nutrition will teach you to eat the right food in order to supply the body with vitamins and the right balance of proteins and carbohydrates that are essential for good health. Achieving the right life-style is not very complicated. The most important thing to remember is that *it's never too late to start.*

 ## A is for attitude

The most important component of a healthy life is a positive attitude. If we understand and accept the fact that we are ourselves largely responsible for how we feel, then we can look at the future without fear. It's possible to enjoy life at an advanced age if we put in a little bit of hard work. If we learn to see difficulties and hardships as challenges, rather than as insurmountable obstacles, we will have come a long way towards having the right attitude to life.

Some people are born with an optimistic and cheerful personality; it is easier for them to look at the future with confidence. It is important, however, for everybody to understand how they can stay young in body and mind, and to *want* to do it. If we keep active by exercising both our body and our mind, we can avoid being a 'burden on society', and perhaps make a contribution to it instead. We can stay interesting and fun to be with, *if* we have the right approach.

 ## E is for effort and exercise

Many negative aspects associated with ageing have more to do with life-style than with actual age. Old people have a tendency to move very little and to sit around most of the day. Physical decline, which is blamed on the ageing process, is more likely to be due to inactivity: people who take no exercise are unfit, stiff and tired, whatever their age. They have bad circulation and low energy levels. Research shows that a physically active person has about a twenty-year advantage in function over a sedentary person: an active 65-year-old has the same physical age as a sedentary 45-year-old.

Regular physical exercise greatly slows down the ageing process. Though we may no longer be able to work our body as hard as when we were young, it is still possible to keep in great shape. There is no need to push ourselves to the point of exhaustion in order to keep fit: regular moderate exercise is enough to make us very fit indeed. If in addition we make sure that we grasp every opportunity to move around in the course of our daily life, we will have both stamina and strength.

Nutrition simply means food

Healthy eating habits are an important part of a healthy life. The benefits of regular exercise go hand in hand with eating those foods that are essential for keeping the body in good shape. We need to eat much less as we age; but we need to eat the right food. An ageing body has specific needs in order to maintain good health. Certain vitamins and minerals are essential to keep old bones strong, maintain muscle strength, and keep the circulation healthy.

Old people often have very bad nutrition, mainly because of lack of information, or low income, or both. A healthy diet is neither expensive nor complicated. Some older people even think they no longer need to try to stick to a healthy diet. They may feel that, as it is boring to be old, they should be allowed to indulge in unhealthy food; they eat for comfort, and have no motivation to try to eat in a healthy way.

Though it is true that many doctors feel that old people need not pay much attention to weight or cholesterol, an unhealthy diet will soon cause health problems, which lead to illness and suffering. Healthy eating makes you feel better. This should be enough to make people want to eat the right things.

Obesity in old age is more life-threatening and uncomfortable than at a younger age. Clinically obese older people are short of breath, tired, and likely to have increasingly aching joints and swollen ankles. This makes them even less inclined to keep active. It can also make them feel depressed.

It is much easier than ever before to maintain a healthy diet. The press is full of nutritional facts and advice, and healthy food is widely available in even the smallest grocery shops. In short, there is no excuse for not eating what you should eat, and it is not boring or difficult. In fact, trying different foods is interesting and exciting. Learning to cook new dishes is also stimulating for the brain; it could be 'food for thought' in more ways than one!

What about our genes?

It is often said that if you want to live to a good old age, you have to choose the right parents. Until quite recently it was believed that as much as 70 per cent of our health circumstances and life expectancy was decided by our genes. This is not so: only about 30 per cent of our physical make-up is genetic, according to recent scientific discoveries. The rest is up to us. That is why we cannot blame our parents, grandparents or old Uncle Joe for the fact that we are unfit, fat, or suffering from certain illnesses. It is mainly our life-style that decides the state of our health. The amount of exercise we take, what we eat, whether we smoke or drink too much alcohol, are far more likely to affect our health than the fact that Granny died of cancer or emphysema.

While modern medicine has made huge improvements in curing many previously life-threatening illnesses, and discovered ways to prolong life for people suffering from incurable ones, it is better to try to avoid becoming ill in the first place. While there is no guarantee, even with an exceptionally healthy life-style, that we will not contract a serious illness, the odds are more favourable if we try to keep healthy. Even if there is a genetic tendency for certain conditions, looking after our health may lessen the suffering, apart from helping us avoid it altogether. In other words, *it is not the cards you are dealt that matter most, it is how you play your hand.*

Staying alert

We must also stimulate our brain. It is only by continuing to learn and use our brain that we can slow down the ageing of our mind. A large part of the decrease in brain function that is considered age-related is actually lack of stimulation. People tend to become more passive as they age, mentally as well as physically. The older we are, the more important it is to keep using our brain. Unfortunately, the reverse is usually the reality: older people often stop trying to learn new skills or acquire information. It is not necessary to do complicated mental gymnastics or to attempt difficult tasks: simple things such as reading or doing crosswords are enough to keep your brain active, provided they are done regularly.

 ## Looking young

There is a tendency in the western world to criticise people because they no longer look young. This 'youth cult' causes unhappiness for many people, especially women, who often start worrying about looking old when they are still in their thirties. They may feel they are worth less because they show their age. Some women spend enormous amounts of money and even suffer terrible pain going through surgery in the hope of keeping a youthful appearance.

Many people are obsessed with age. They always want to know how old people are, and if they don't know they try to guess. 'She must be at least fifty-five,' they say, or 'He doesn't look a day over forty.' It seems so important to put people into a category, so that they can be judged simply on the basis of their age. It's the same in the press. 'Woman (45) rides bareback across the Himalayas,' we read. Her age is the first thing we need to know before we can assess her fantastic achievement!

Nobody loves grey hair, wrinkles, or the sight of a sagging body. But is it not time to fight against this prejudice? It's impossible to look twenty-five for ever, even with the most advanced plastic surgery. More than half the world's population are over fifty. In twenty years' time, more people will be old than young. The majority will look old, with wrinkles and grey hair. It's quite absurd to think that we must all have smooth skin to be acceptable to each other!

We should try to look *well* rather than young. If we have good health—and that includes a reasonable level of fitness—we will look attractive. A healthy body and a positive attitude make anybody look great, never mind their age! Someone who has plenty of interests and a zest for life is wonderful company, at any age. Young or old, we are always drawn to people who are full of enthusiasm and energy.

Feeling young

Young people do not feel young—they feel normal. Older people say they feel young when they feel well. Some people are lucky enough to feel well most of the time. Perhaps it is not luck but good health achieved by the right life-style.

Feeling young also depends on our attitude to life. A forty-year-old may feel older than an eighty-year-old, because he or she is worried about the signs of ageing and the prospect of growing older. The eighty-year-old may have accepted looking older and may simply be delighted to feel well enough to do the things he or she enjoys. If we can forget about our age and get on with living, growing older is easier to bear. Everything is relative: it all depends on what we are comparing ourselves with. If we compare ourselves at sixty with how we felt at twenty, we will feel very old indeed. It depends on what we think is normal at the age we are. If we feel exceptionally well at sixty but have the idea that we should feel old and tired at that age, we will think of ourselves as 'young for our age.'

Feeling young or old stems from our attitude to ourselves, and to life in general. If we have confidence in ourselves and see no limits to what we can achieve, age does not matter a great deal. People often restrict their activities to what they believe they should be able to do at a certain age. Retirement often creates this kind of thinking. When people retire, they may feel that they have to stop not only their working life but a lot of their leisure activities as well. 'Retirement' is itself a negative word: it gives the idea that we somehow 'retire' from life and enter another world, the world of those who are no longer an important part of society. It should be a period in our lives when we can spend more time doing things that are enjoyable, things we were too busy to do when we were working full time.

Retired people can be extremely useful in their community. They can help look after people who live on their own, be active in local politics, or help collect money for charity. Helping others is a wonderful way to get to know people, and it is the best way to feel young. By helping others we forget our own problems and perhaps learn that there are people worse off than ourselves. Many old people who live alone would love to have someone visit them for a chat, to read them the newspaper, or walk their dog. We don't have to look very hard to find somebody who would like company from time to time: every community has plenty of people who live alone and are lonely. It may not be the most fun you ever had, but helping an old woman with her garden, or her shopping, or even tidying up the kitchen, will earn you her heartfelt thanks. Mixing good deeds with enjoyable activities is very satisfying. You can then indulge yourself with a good conscience. The time may come when you will need help yourself!

'Supergran'

My mother, who is in her late seventies, told me that she is at her best when she is so busy that she doesn't have time to think about how she feels. Her idea of 'gardening' is cutting down a tree, dragging it to the other end of the garden, and cutting it up with a chain-saw. She is not a freak of nature but an example of how we should all be, even at an advanced age.

There is a type of old person who is youthful and healthy in old age. We all meet them from time to time: the eighty-year-old who walks five miles every day, plays tennis or golf regularly, and travels all over the world; the ninety-year-old who rides horses and swims fifty lengths without a bother; the 95-year-old who still looks after the garden and walks the dogs. My own grandmother, who lived to 104, went to language classes in her nineties, exercised until she was well over a hundred, and read at least a chapter of a novel every day until the last year of her life. (She particularly liked *The Three Musketeers*.) We see these people as somehow miraculous, and talk about them as if they have supernatural powers. They haven't. They simply have that extra drive, vitality, 'get up and go,' or whatever you would like to call it. They never lose their enthusiasm or curiosity.

These 'young' old people are not spared the stiffness and discomfort of an ageing body. They simply ignore the aches and pains, probably because it is so important to them to be able to do the things they enjoy. Their will to keep active helps them overcome their physical deficiencies.

I regularly go horse-riding with a man who has recently celebrated his eightieth birthday. I was impressed to see him ride his horse at full gallop and jump a big obstacle. 'Do you often think about your age?' I asked him. 'All the time,' he replied. I had assumed that, since he was able to ride in a way that would be daunting to someone half his age, he didn't feel in any way weak. The answer is that he *does* feel his age, but his wish to do things is stronger than the fear of pain. 'My mind decides what I want to do, and my body just has to do its best to follow,' he explained. Mind over matter, in other words.

Aches and pains

As we age, we have to get used to the fact that life is more difficult. The body of an older person does not function as well as a that of a twenty-year-old. We often have to 'kick-start' ourselves in the morning; there is a certain stiffness in joints and muscles, and many physical activities leave their mark in the form of fatigue and discomfort (and that's already at around the age of fifty!). The secret is not to 'feel' so much, and to keep going despite the minor twinges. Pacing ourselves is also important. We have to realise that we cannot keep up with younger people when it comes to many sports; but this should not be a reason to become passive. Even if we no longer have the same speed and strength as before, it doesn't mean we have none at all. Older people can maintain great strength and stamina, with regular exercise.

Many older people are convinced that they suffer from arthritis because they feel stiff at times. It is often simply muscle strain from some unaccustomed exercise, or doing housework or gardening. Many supposed arthritis sufferers have in fact rheumatism, which is a different ailment altogether. (See chapter 8.) It is important to have regular medical check-ups to ascertain the cause of pain and discomfort.

Conclusion

'Old age is fifteen years older than I am,' says a friend (twenty years older than me). He also says there are three stages in life: young, middle-aged, and 'you're looking very well!'

Growing old mainly happens in our minds. We often think of ourselves as old long before anybody else does. But if you believe you are young, you will probably appear a lot younger than you are. If you are determined to keep going and to accept the fact that you are growing older, ageing will not be the great tragedy many people fear. After all, we are the same person we have always been, even though there is an older man or woman looking out at us from the mirror.

A healthy life-style gives confidence, dignity, and independence. Staying healthy as long as possible will ensure that we can cope with life without the help of others. Society will have to cope with a huge number of old people in the future. Imagine the expense of looking after a vast ageing population that is generally unwell! The present generation have fewer children than the previous one, but they will have another burden to carry: us. Our children will not thank us for having to foot the bill for our health care—but perhaps that is one way to pay them back for sleepless nights, teenage tantrums, and college fees!

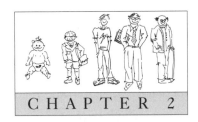

CHAPTER 2

A LONGER SHELF LIFE
HOW TO SLOW DOWN THE AGEING PROCESS

We start to age from the moment we are born. Ageing in the physiological sense, however, starts around the age of twenty. Up to that point, changes in the body are part of natural development and growth. 'Ageing' starts from the moment the functions of our various organs begin to slowly deteriorate. How, and at what rate, this deterioration takes place depends partly on hereditary factors, partly on our life-style.

In this chapter I explain what happens to our bodies as we age, what we can expect at a certain age, how the different parts of our body change with time, and to what extent a healthy life can slow down the ageing process.

From birth to old age

❭ 0–14

This is a period of enormous growth. We learn to sit, crawl, stand, walk, run, and jump. Girls are born with a smaller but more developed brain than boys, and their skeleton is also more developed at birth. They develop finer motor skills earlier than boys; but boys spend longer developing the larger movements, such as jumping and running.

⟩ Puberty

This stage is marked by the onset of periods, the start of the development of breasts and increased fat layers (by 15–25 per cent) for girls, and by beard growth, increased muscle mass and a deeper voice for boys.

Girls generally grow until the beginning of puberty, the moment they start having periods. Boys do not grow very tall before puberty but then have a huge surge in growth around the age of fourteen to sixteen. At this stage boys overtake girls in both height and weight. Our bodies work hard to grow and develop.

⟩ 15–25

This is the period during which we are most alive. By the age of twenty our weight has increased twenty times. Our fertility, strength and speed are at their optimum; our capacity to take in oxygen is at its peak. Our maximum pulse rate (the highest pulse rate measured in connection with the greatest effort of the large muscle groups) is about 200 beats a minute.

A woman's monthly cycle has stabilised, and her hormone levels are well balanced.

The average male will have twice the strength of a woman. Strength per muscle cell is the same for women as for men, but women have more 'slow' fibres, which give stamina but less strength. Men may have greater precision when it comes to shooting and throwing a ball, but women have better co-ordination when it comes to movements (dancing and gymnastics). People keen on competition in sports have the greatest chance of succeeding at the age of twenty to twenty-five. Bodies have stabilised and found their balance.

⟩ 25–40

The skeleton strengthens until the age of thirty-five, then it becomes weaker. Women lose 1 per cent of their bone mass per year (2 to 6 per cent during menopause). Our ligaments begin to age at around twenty-five. In fact all organs start to decline during this period. The impulses in the nerve cells diminish, and we don't move as fast as when we were younger. This is also because our breathing is not as effective as before and the heart no longer has the capacity it used to have to pump blood around the body. Muscle mass decreases and becomes less elastic. The maximum pulse rate is lower.

40–55

From forty onwards the brain loses 2 to 3 grams in weight per year. Our metabolism slows down, making it more difficult to keep a slim figure. Our arteries and blood vessels harden, and the muscle cells of the heart begin to weaken. The first wrinkles become apparent, and loss of elasticity in the skin combined with the force of gravity makes our bodies sag. Our stomach and bottom want to hang down.

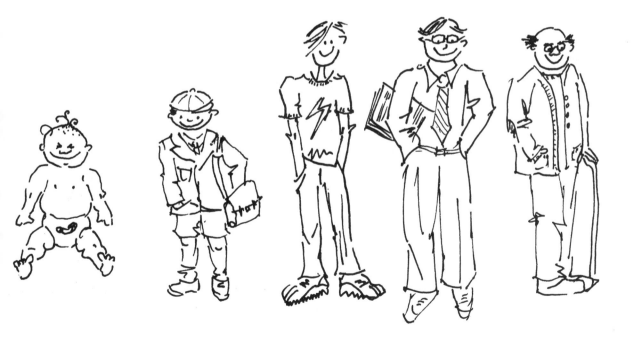

The skin's cells do not renew themselves as quickly as before. The muscles of our eyes lose elasticity, and we need glasses to read. Some men have thinning hair.

Women usually go through the menopause at this age. Diminishing levels of oestrogen cause a number of problems, notably thinning bones, 'hot flushes', and mood swings. Heart and circulation problems are more common at this age than before, because the arteries become less elastic as we age. Men around the age of fifty who are overweight have a high risk of heart disease.

❱ 55–65

This is when most people realise finally that they are ageing. We notice more wrinkles, our hair is greying, and changes in the pigment in our skin may give us 'age spots' (brown spots that are mostly caused by overexposure to sunlight). The whites of our eyes, teeth and nails become more yellow. A woman at this age can have lost as much as a third of her original bone mass.

The impulses between nerve cells are slower, which causes diminished speed and suppleness in our movements. Bone fractures are more and more common as we age, because our bones become more brittle. Back problems, such as a slipped disc, can easily occur because of increased stiffness in the lower lumbar region.

❱ 65–75 and beyond

We start to experience more of the problems associated with old age at about seventy-five. We have less muscle fibre, our bones are even more brittle, and our ligaments and tendons become hard and stiff. Injuries such as hip fractures are common in women after seventy-five; hip replacements may be necessary. We start to look physically older, with weaker tendons and muscles in the neck and back resulting in a stooping posture. The hips are stiffer, and we may find it hard to stretch out our legs, which can make walking difficult.

How to slow down ageing

Our bodies deteriorate the older we get; but the speed at which this process takes place depends on many things. As only 30 per cent of our general health is due to heredity, how can we age better and more slowly? What can we do, and at what age? There are certain measures we can take at different stages in our life.

❱ In our thirties

This is the age at which we can begin to lay down the foundation of a healthy old age. As we start losing bone mass at about thirty-five, it is important to take up weight-bearing exercise, to get aerobically fit, and to pay attention to a healthy diet.

❱ The right strategy at this age

Your body is at its peak when it comes to strength and stamina, so this is the time to sample some new sports, if you haven't been very active before. A mixture of jogging, aerobics, cycling, tennis, squash or weight-training three to four times a week will work your heart and lungs, strengthen your bones, and trim your body.

If the demands of work and family are making it hard to stick to a regular exercise routine, sign up for an exercise class. It is a good investment in your mental and physical health, and it may provide the extra incentive you need to stay strong. Taking the stairs every chance you get and carrying your bags at the supermarket or the airport will squeeze some bone-strengthening into your day when you can't get to the gym.

If you are a woman, a bone scan in your late thirties will show any deficiency in bone mass. As it is still possible to build up diminishing bone up to the age of forty-five, finding out the state of your bones at this stage is very important. If there is a family history of osteoporosis, you should be especially vigilant.

When it comes to diet, try to cut down on fat and increase your intake of calcium (800 mg a day at this age), and make sure you eat a *minimum* of five helpings of fruit and vegetables a day.

This is the time to stop smoking. A few years after you stop, your health will be nearly as good as if you had never smoked.

Using sun block and trying to stay out of strong sunshine will protect your skin from premature ageing, and protect you from skin cancer.

Six rules to stick to in your thirties

1. Have a bone scan (especially if you are a woman).
2. Increase the amount of calcium in your diet.
3. Start taking regular weight-bearing exercise.
4. Stop smoking.
5. Stay out of the sun.
6. Increase your daily consumption of fruit and vegetables.

In your forties

At this age you may find that keeping your shape is suddenly more difficult, even if you are a sports fanatic. We lose about a third of a pound of muscle a year around forty, and gain about the same in fat. Twinges in knees or back are painful souvenirs of running in bad shoes, or lifting small children. A few grey hairs begin to show. Is this the beginning of a physical decline?

What to do at this stage

There is no need to worry about a few grey hairs and the odd twinge at this age; adding a little weight-lifting, extra gardening or housework to your day can give you back the firm body you remember. Building muscle also increases your metabolism: you can increase it by as much as 15 per cent if you lift weights or do other strengthening exercises three times a week. Muscles burn more calories than fat. For the average-sized person, this means burning an extra 300 calories a day.

Dieting alone is not a healthy option, because it will make you lose muscle, bone and other lean tissue with the fat.

There is no need to join a gym or buy expensive exercise equipment: a few light weights can be bought in any sports shop, and with the help of an exercise video or instructions from a book you can organise your own work-outs.

If you have never exercised, it is still possible to take up quite vigorous activities, such as jogging, high-impact aerobics, squash, or singles tennis, provided you check with your doctor and start any new exercise or sport gradually.

If you are nervous about how your knees or other achy joints will respond to increased training, take heart from new studies that prove that exercise is the best treatment for osteo-arthritis (see chapter 8). Keeping active can prevent arthritis from getting worse and may ensure a pain-free old age.

Regular exercise has also been shown to improve mild depression, so common among the elderly. It may even remove the need for antidepressant drugs in some cases.

You will notice a certain deterioration in your sight at this age. Suddenly it is difficult to see small type in books and newspapers; some texts have to be held at arm's length to be seen clearly. The muscles of your eyes are losing their elasticity, and you will need reading glasses. Make an appointment with an eye specialist for a check-up (an optician is not competent to perform all the tests necessary for a thorough examination). From now on, a once-yearly check-up of your eyes is important to ensure good vision and prevent small problems becoming more serious.

Women close to the menopause should seek the advice of a gynaecologist about possible menopausal problems and discuss the option of taking hormones. You should also have your heart, blood pressure and cholesterol level checked (this applies to men as well), as diminishing hormone levels mean less protection from heart disease.

If you have not had a bone scan, have one now. Increase your daily intake of calcium to 1,200 mg, and make sure you fit in some weight-bearing exercise at least three times a week. (This is beneficial for men as well.)

It is also important to make sure you improve your memory and stimulate your brain at this age. Learning something new or improving existing skills, such as languages, computer skills, or taking up a new hobby, are good ways to activate the brain cells and make sure you don't lose too many of them. (See chapter 3.)

❯ In your forties you should

~ make sure you mix strength training with weight-bearing exercise

~ stimulate your mind by learning something new

~ have a bone scan

~ increase the calcium in your diet

~ have your eyes checked

~ if you are a woman, see a gynaecologist

~ have your heart, blood pressure and cholesterol level checked

~ cut down on fat in your diet.

❯ In our fifties

This can be a difficult age, as stress at work is combined with worry about children or elderly parents. You may be starting a new career, or thinking about retiring. There could also be disappointments about lost opportunities, relationships gone wrong, or diminishing career breaks. Your body is ageing more noticeably: there is stiffness in joints and muscles in the mornings, and if you are a woman you have problems with menopausal symptoms.

From a health point of view, your body is more fragile now. It is more sensitive to abuse in the form of too much stress at work, late nights, too much alcohol, unhealthy food, or not enough exercise. For women, heart disease becomes a bigger threat after the menopause, along with osteoporosis. Wear and tear on joints and muscles from too much or the wrong type of exercise can make you stiff and sore.

What to do to feel well in your fifties

At this age you should exercise as much as before, but more gently. Walking instead of jogging, and switching from high-impact to low-impact aerobics (where there is no jumping) are good tactics; it will still exercise your muscles, bones and joints without jarring.

If you have not exercised before but want to start, walking is the best way to get your body used to more activity. Start slowly, walking for ten minutes, increasing by five minutes each time, until you are walking for a minimum of thirty minutes three times a week. Other types of aerobic exercise that are good at this age include swimming and cycling—but remember, they are not weight-bearing and will not make your bones stronger. Sports such as tennis and badminton are weight-bearing, but if you take up such a sport for the first time at this age, stick to doubles!

Try to accumulate at least forty-five minutes of moderate aerobic exercise, or thirty minutes of more intense activity, every day for the sake of your heart. There are many things you could do: garden for forty-five minutes, rake leaves, wash windows or floors, walk two miles, or cycle five miles, in half an hour. Swim laps for twenty minutes, or dance for thirty. Even housework and just walking around the house, especially if it includes walking up and down stairs many times a day, qualify as physical activity. Active minutes add up quickly, and they all count.

Stretching, yoga or other moderate activities will strengthen your muscles, make your joints supple, and improve both your balance and your co-ordination. These more gentle activities are excellent for making you relax, which is a great help during times of stress.

If you cannot get to a class, buy a video or book of yoga or stretching for beginners and do it at home.

Regular medical check-ups to make sure your heart and circulation are working well are essential at this age. Take time for hobbies that include mental stimulation, such as bridge, chess, language classes, or learning computer skills. Relax by seeing friends and family more often.

❯ Good ways to stay in great shape in your fifties

~ Exercising regularly but gently

~ Improving co-ordination and balance

~ Relaxing with yoga, stretching, or meditation

~ Keeping an eye on your heart, circulation, and cholesterol levels

~ Stimulating your brain

~ Keeping alcohol levels down

~ Making sure you get enough sleep

~ Taking more time off to see friends and family

~ Eating healthy food

❯ In your sixties

Retirement becomes a reality, and you have to prepare for a different life. At this age we have more time to ourselves. From a health point of view, we become aware of the limitations of an ageing body. We are more vulnerable to infection, as the immune system is weakening. Our memory seems to fail us from time to time, and we are faced with hardships such as bereavement, loneliness, and illness.

❯ How to stay strong in your sixties

A diet rich in vitamins, plenty of exercise and lower levels of stress will keep you in good shape at this stage of your life. Even if you didn't run marathons or spend hours in the gym when you were younger and have always preferred poetry to push-ups, you can still enjoy the benefits of an active life if you start moving now. Studies have shown that at sixty you can increase your muscle strength by 75 per cent, and even slightly increase your bone density. Aerobic exercise will make your heart stronger and keep your blood pressure at a healthy level; it will also boost a weak immune system. One study revealed that people of sixty, seventy and eighty who walked thirty minutes a day, five days a week, spent half as many days a year nursing symptoms of colds as their inactive peers.

Again, walking is the ideal activity, especially for the previously inactive person. Swimming and cycling are also excellent. Yoga and stretching are wonderful for improving muscle strength, flexibility, co-ordination, and balance. As osteo-arthritis affects us more, putting joints through their full range of motion will prevent further pain and stiffness. As I mentioned before, it is not necessary to join a gym (though going to a class is a good way to meet people), as there are so many books and exercise videos on the market these days.

You should include some upper-body strengthening at this age to prevent the stooped posture so common in older people. Lifting light weights will protect your vertebrae from compression fractures—the small cracks that can lead to the curved back known as 'dowager's hump'. Go to a gym and ask an instructor to give you a routine that involves lifting dumbbells. Then you can do it at home with weights bought at a sports shop.

It is more important than ever to exercise our brain cells at this age with plenty of activities such as reading, card games, learning, and memorising.

Any health problems should be dealt with at once, and regular visits to your GP are essential.

⟩ Six healthy habits for the over-sixties

1. Eat foods rich in vitamins to boost the immune system.
2. Never spend a day without some kind of exercise.
3. 'Pump some iron' to keep your back straight.
4. Stretch your mind with games, books, puzzles, and quizzes.
5. Keep supple with stretching or other gentle exercise.
6. Do something you enjoy every day.

❭ Your seventies, eighties, and nineties

This is the age when we reap the benefits of an active life. If you have exercised or practised sports all your life, you will be in excellent health and probably appear years younger than your actual age. Keep going! There is no need to put away the tennis racket, running-shoes, or golf clubs; you don't have to get off the horse or stop cycling. You may find that you have to slow down the pace somewhat, and you are probably a little stiffer. That is not a reason to stop, however.

If you have spent your younger years as a couch potato, don't worry. You can still take up exercise and greatly improve your health and fitness; but in that case you must consult your doctor first, and start slowly. Walking and swimming are the best activities to take up for previously sedentary people. Yoga and stretching are also good. Golf, doubles tennis and badminton are good sports to learn, as they also stimulate your brain and improve co-ordination and balance. It all depends on the type of thing you enjoy and what you can afford.

At this age, women are often affected by osteoporosis, and hip fractures are common. Ageing hearts and blood circulation can make high blood pressure more prevalent. Osteo-arthritis makes joints and muscles stiff and sore. The immune system is weaker, and you may be more susceptible to colds and flu symptoms.

A healthy diet is particularly important now. Follow the example of people in the countries around the Mediterranean and eat plenty of fish, fruit, vegetables, and olive oil. Add more fibre in the form of whole-wheat bread or cereal, which will help your digestive system. It is vitally important to include plenty of fibre in your diet, as older people are more susceptible to constipation and more serious problems that can follow as a result. A glass of wine or other spirits a day is beneficial for the heart and blood circulation, but more than two drinks a day could have the opposite effect. If you like a drink, try to stick to a maximum of two a day.

Try not to sit still for too long, as that will make you stiff and numb. Keep your circulation going by moving around a little every half an hour when you are watching television.

Stretch your mind by thinking, learning, reading, and listening.

Follow the example of old people in America, who have the habit of having a complete medical check-up every year. That way they monitor their health and nip minor problems in the bud, before they become more serious.

Older people are more sensitive to cold. In the winter, make sure you have at least one room in the house at a comfortable temperature; and wear warm clothes, a hat and gloves when you go outside.

Make sure you get at least fifteen minutes' sun or daylight on your skin (your face or hands) every day in order to get the benefit of vitamin D.

How to be energetic at eighty

~ Do some kind of physical activity for at least half an hour every day.

~ Pretend you are Greek, and eat what they do.

~ Look after your bones by including enough calcium in your diet, and combine it with some weight-bearing exercise.

~ Eat plenty of fibre.

~ Have a drink or two each day, but no more.

~ Don't sit still for long periods.

~ Exercise your mind.

~ See your doctor at least once a year.

~ Stay warm.

~ Go outdoors for half an hour or more every day.

Perhaps you could follow the example of Helen, a woman I read about recently. Three years ago her husband died of cancer. About the same time, a new gym opened in her locality. 'It saved my life,' she said. 'I made myself get up and go.' Though she and her husband had walked together a few times a week, Helen had never been very active. Now she walks regularly and goes to the gym five times a week. She uses the treadmill, the stationary bike, the rowing machine, and the weight machine, and she stretches. She has acquired an agility she never thought possible; she has a lot of energy and feels great. Helen is eighty-three.

Staying in touch

The senses—vision, hearing, smell, taste, and touch—are our communication system with the world around us. Loss or deterioration of some of our senses, such as hearing and vision, may occur with age or because of our activities: repeated loud noise can lead to hearing loss; eye damage can be the result of exposure to sunlight. Diabetes can be a factor in certain types of eye problems.

❭ The eyes

Apart from needing glasses to read, there are other problems that can affect the older person's eyesight, such as cataracts, glaucoma, and macular degeneration.

Cataracts are a more serious condition that can develop as you age. A cataract is a clouding of the lens of the eye, preventing light passing through. If the clouded area of the lens is at the side rather than in the middle, you can probably live with it, as it will not interfere greatly with your vision; but if it stops you reading, driving, or enjoying life in general, consider surgery. It is the only way to treat cataracts, and it is simple: you can even have it done as an outpatient. Most people have the cataract removed and an artificial lens inserted. If you need surgery on both eyes, they are usually treated a few weeks or months apart. Cataract surgery usually has dramatic results, giving many people a new lease of life.

Glaucoma is a serious condition in which the internal pressure of the eye increases, and if it is not treated it can result in blindness. In a normal eye, a fluid called the *aqueous humour* flows from the middle part of the eye, around the lens and into the front part, then back through a special drainage system around the edge of the iris. In glaucoma the drainage system is partially or totally blocked, increasing the pressure within the eye and eventually damaging the optic nerve.

Glaucoma is usually treated with eye drops that dilate the drainage system, decreasing the pressure. The problem with glaucoma is that it has almost no symptoms. There is no pain, and the first sign is usually a partial loss of vision.

Macular degeneration is a condition that affects the *retina,* the thin film lining the back of the eye that receives images. The *macula* is the central part of the retina where the lens focuses an image. In macular degeneration this part of the retina breaks down, resulting in blurred vision or even partial blindness. About 70 per cent of macular degeneration is due to ageing, and the rest is caused by disease, infection, or accidents. An eye specialist can detect it early. It can be treated with lasers, and there is also some research that suggests that including vitamin E in our diet may help prevent the disease.

It is important to visit an eye specialist regularly as we grow older in order to have the pressure in our eyes checked and to detect the early signs of disease. An optician can fit you with glasses and check your vision but cannot treat medical problems or carry out tests for diseases. Only a doctor can deal with serious problems.

The ears

Loss of hearing is one of the most common signs of ageing, yet many old people refuse to admit that they do not hear very well. About 30 per cent of all people between the ages of sixty-five and seventy-five have some hearing loss, and 50 per cent of people over seventy-five. If we refuse to admit that our hearing is deteriorating it can make us appear senile or forgetful. If people around us are aware that we have trouble hearing, they will make sure we hear important things, and we will not miss vital information.

Don't be embarrassed about using a hearing aid, as it can make a huge difference to your life. Many people need glasses; so think of a hearing aid as a similar object.

There are a number of different kinds of hearing aids on the market today, and they are becoming more and more advanced. There are also devices for the television, called caption decoders, that put dialogue in the form of text at the bottom of the screen, rather like sub-titles.

❭ Taste and smell

Some older people lose some of their ability to taste and smell. This is not in itself debilitating, but it may interfere with the enjoyment of food. It may show up first as a loss of appetite, which could lead to malnutrition. If you feel you have lost some of your ability to taste or smell, you must see a doctor. There are some reversible conditions that give rise to these symptoms: it may simply be a case of blocked sinuses, which can be cleared up with the right medication.

Looking after your teeth is also important for the enjoyment of food. Bad teeth can interfere with chewing and digestion, as well as being unsightly. Losing your teeth is not inevitable as you age but rather the result of poor dental hygiene. Daily brushing and flossing and twice-yearly dental check-ups will ensure that your teeth stay healthy and where they belong: in your mouth.

Living longer

The question of longevity and why some people live to a very old age is still a mystery. It is widely assumed that a long life is due to genes and that having relatives who lived to a very old age will ensure that we will do the same. As I pointed out earlier, this has been found to be largely untrue. Life expectancy is not inherited, like blood groups. If you have exceptionally long-lived parents you still cannot take longevity for granted.

Variation of life-span is mostly linked to life-style. Nutrition is important: a poor diet—high in saturated fats and sugar—can shorten life. On the other hand, eating a lot of vegetables, fish and soya products appears to be beneficial, which may explain why the Japanese are the longest-lived nation in the world. Exercise, low stress levels, avoiding tobacco and a low intake of alcohol are additional factors thought to increase life-span.

The effects of a healthy life-style on ageing have been known by health professionals for some time. It is now generally agreed that how we age is not something we have been 'programmed' with: instead, it is decided by the accumulation during our lifetime of insidious little faults in the tissues and cells of our body. How long we live is decided by a balance between how fast things go wrong within our cells and how diligently they work to prevent damage building up.

In addition to life-style and genes, there is a third factor that decides how we age: chance. Even in the animal world, the difference between individuals with the same genes and living conditions is often great. Some are lucky, while others are not. This variation in health between genetically identical individuals can be observed in twins, who may develop very different age-related diseases. That is why we must not consider old people to be the same. All seventy-year-olds are not identical: some may be healthier than people ten years younger, while others could feel, and appear, many years older than their chronological age.

Not only do we live longer today than before but, because of improved living conditions, we are also in better shape at an older age. We must do our best to keep up this trend.

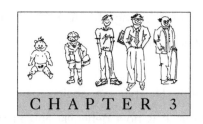

CHAPTER 3

WAKE UP YOUR MIND
HOW TO KEEP YOUR MIND ACTIVE

The brain is the most important part of the body in the battle against ageing. Apart from the fact that it is a mysterious, amazing and wonderful organ, which controls everything we do, think, and feel, it also decides how we age.

It is generally believed that our brain slowly deteriorates as we age. Loss of memory, lack of co-ordination and poor perception are all supposed to come with age, and most people think that these disabilities are inevitable. While it is true that the brain starts losing cells from about the age of thirty and there is a certain loss of elasticity, much of the decline is due to lack of stimulation rather than to age.

A certain degree of forgetfulness *is* inevitable as we age; but more important functions of the mind, such as imagination and creativity, are mostly unaffected by ageing. We may forget where we put the keys, the name of someone we met at a party, or what we went upstairs to get, but we are still able to enjoy a good book, beautiful music, and fine art. We can form new friendships, and fall in love, until we die. Many famous artists were still hard at work into old age, sometimes producing their best work late in their lives. Some scientists made their most important discoveries when they were well over the age at which most people retire.

There are many ways in which our behaviour throughout life influences how we age. Our attitude to life, the amount of exercise we take, our diet and the extent to which we have indulged in an unhealthy life-style all have an effect on the brain as we grow older; but most important of all is the amount of stimulation we give it.

The best way to ensure that the brain does not lose too many of its functions as we age is to *use* it. 'Use it or lose it,' it is sometimes said of the muscles; and it is the same with the brain. It is essential to stimulate our mind every day of our lives if we don't want to experience a great deal of memory loss and lack of intellectual capacity later.

Young at heart

People who age well, look young and are fit and healthy in mind and body well into an advanced age all have a positive attitude. More often than not this is due to their inherited personality—something they are born with. It can also be the way they were brought up, and the example their parents gave to them. Someone who was constantly told as a child not to fuss about minor problems and never to give up is likely to have learnt from an early age to cope with problems.

Some people don't seem to worry too much about the fact that they both look and feel older; they don't seem to notice that they have aged, and continue their lives much as before. They even seem to enjoy having more time to travel, or to pursue hobbies. Many of them embark on a new career or begin to learn a new skill. They are highly adaptable and open to new ideas.

When we are older we can acquire knowledge for its own sake, rather than to advance our careers. You may always have wanted to learn about the Incas, or how to play the piano. Now is your chance. If you have a lot of time on your hands because you are retired from your job and the children have moved out, use it to learn something new. It is never a waste of time or effort. You can learn languages, computer skills, history, art or science, a craft, or how to play a musical instrument. The list is endless.

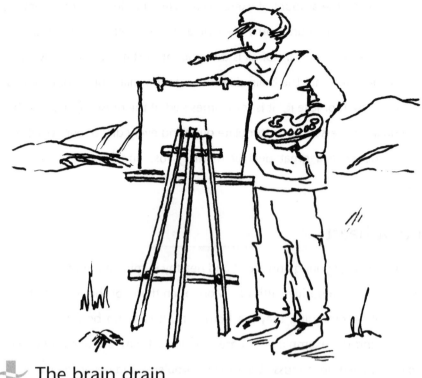

The brain drain

It is widely believed that we lose brain cells at an alarming rate as we age. Recent studies, however, show that it is not as bad as was previously thought. The results of research using both human and monkey brains indicate that most of the cells that make up the *neocortex,* the part of the brain used for thinking, survive well into our seventies. The myth of the dying brain was a result of earlier studies that included victims of Alzheimer's disease and other dementia sufferers. Alzheimer's disease was not as well diagnosed in the early post-war years, when the first studies took place, and some of its milder symptoms were accepted as part of normal ageing.

While it is true that the brain shrinks slightly as we age, this shrinkage does not happen in the grey matter, which contains all the 'thinking parts' of the brain. The grey matter is situated in the *cerebral cortex,* that stuff that looks like a pickled walnut. Exercising your mind with puzzles, games and other activities that make you think hard actually thickens the grey matter. The *frontal lobe*—the front of the pickled walnut—is the part where your personality is; any damage to this part can result in dramatic personality changes.

The latest research shows that the decline in mental function as we age results from a breakdown in the *myelin,* the fatty sheath that surrounds the core of the nerve fibre that conducts impulses from cells. Myelin enables messages to be transmitted throughout the network of the brain. If the myelin sheath breaks down, the nerve cells become exposed and the network is no longer as efficient as before. People who have amazing mental powers in old age may have a genetic predisposition that protects the myelin sheath from breaking down; but they are probably using their brain by keeping mentally active as well.

There is great hope for those who do not have such a genetic advantage. New medication may soon be available that can prevent the myelin from deteriorating.

Mental gymnastics

The only way to maintain our intellectual capacity is to use our brain. If the mind is stimulated every day of our lives, it will stay reasonably alert. We can even increase the brain's ability to accept information in this way. Like muscles, the brain will atrophy if it is not used. Muscles can be built up again, even after a long period of non-use; but it is not possible to rescue lost brain cells.

It is not as difficult and complicated as it sounds. Simple activities are enough, provided they make you think. Reading, writing and solving puzzles are just some examples of mental gymnastics.

A recent experiment using rats illustrates this fact. Three groups of rats were given different environments. The first group had a cage full of playthings, such as ladders, ramps, and wheels, giving them plenty of opportunity to entertain themselves. The second group had no toys but were allowed to watch the first group. The third group had no toys and nothing to watch. Not surprisingly, the first group of rats was found to have better brain capacity than the other two. You might expect the second group, the one that was allowed to watch the first group, to score higher than the rats that had nothing to do or to watch, but these two groups scored almost equally badly. The conclusion is that it is not enough to have a visually stimulating environment: our minds must be actively stimulated in order to be kept alert.

Mental exercise is as important for the brain as physical exercise is for the body. Even things like saying the alphabet backwards, trying to find as many words as possible starting with the same letter or memorising other lists are good methods for 'flexing' your brain.

Games such as bridge, chess and Scrabble are enjoyable, stimulate the memory, and greatly exercise the brain. Trivial Pursuit is an excellent game for working your memory.

Reading books and newspapers, listening to the radio and watching television, while not actually exercising the brain, are stimulating because they provide information and are enjoyable and distracting. Doing something you enjoy and learning about the world through the media are important as we grow older. You will always have something to talk about by staying in touch with what happens around you. But you also have to do something that makes you think and remember every day.

Painting, drawing, writing and singing are all creative pastimes and very good activities for the brain. Cooking, sewing (especially embroidery) and gardening can also be described as creative. DIY and even housework that involves making your house look nice and welcoming qualify as well.

Change is also stimulating. Taking a different route on your daily walk, reading a different paper, moving the furniture around or even changing your hairstyle or clothes are all ways to make your daily routine more lively. It is boring to stick to the same pattern always, and boredom is bad for our mental health.

Keeping in touch

Another way to stimulate the mind is social interaction. Meeting people and discussing common interests, politics or the latest gossip is important for everybody. It has been found that people who are described as gregarious have greater mental capacity than those who are loners.

As we grow older we have to make greater efforts to mix with others. Join a club, a sewing circle, a committee—or start your own. How about starting a reading group, where you read a book and meet regularly to discuss it? Invite your friends and neighbours for a cup of tea. Ask at your local church if they need help with flowers or other chores. Invite your family to visit often. Walk the dog in the park and meet other dog-owners. We all have hobbies and interests, and with a little effort we can meet people who share them.

 How to improve your memory

There are two types of memory: short-term (what we are thinking about right now), and long-term (our permanent data-base). One of the first signs of declining brain function as we age is the deterioration of our short-term memory. This can start to happen as early as our forties. Suddenly we cannot remember people's names as easily as before; the car keys are mislaid and then found in a place we have no recollection of having put them; phone numbers seem impossible to memorise; and learning anything is more difficult than before.

This is only partly due to ageing. The older we are, the more responsibilities and concerns we have in our lives. Young people have only themselves to worry about and can spend all their time concentrating on learning, which of course includes memorising. Older people have many worries and duties to tackle each day, making it harder to keep information fresh in their minds.

It is also a question of priorities. Many things we 'forget' we have probably not taken in properly because we didn't concentrate on them in the first place. It may not have seemed important, or we were distracted by something else. People who seem to have an impressive memory for names are probably interested in meeting others and love to find out things about them; those who confess to 'being terrible with names' are probably just not interested in meeting other people. If we make a conscious effort to retain information, such as names and numbers, our minds will not be a total blank when we try to retrieve it.

Memory is also a matter of training. If you get into the habit of imprinting information on your mind, you will soon find that you can remember a lot more than before.

Next time you meet someone new, try to imprint his or her name in your mind by using an image. Look at the person's face, and repeat the name. Try to associate the name with an image. John Smith could be 'Blacksmith', Liz Jones 'Whiz Phones', or Jane Mulligan 'Vain Hooligan'. Repeat the name to yourself a few times (the real one, or you may call the person something embarrassing the next time!). Ten minutes later, repeat the real name and the association in your mind. I can guarantee that you will not forget that name.

We use our short-term memory to remember a phone number. It will usually stay in our mind long enough only for us to write it down; to imprint it into our long-term memory we have to repeat it over and over again. A number we use often can be remembered without consulting the telephone book.

One way to imprint numbers in your mind is to translate them into letters or words that have a meaning for you. For example, 24448 could be translated into 'Tom fast, fast, fast ate.' Try finding words that give a meaning to something in your life. The more exaggerated and comic, the better.

If you tell yourself out loud where you put down your key or your glasses, you will not lose them. Say, 'I'm putting the car keys on the hall table,' for example. You may seem a bit eccentric, but not forgetful!

Choose a short poem, a saying, a Bible verse or a sentence from a newspaper article and try to memorise it. Repeat it over and over again for several minutes;

then leave it and come back to it later, repeating it a few times again. Do this several times a week, and you will find your memory greatly improved.

As it is the short-term memory that causes most problems, we should try to imprint as much as possible into our long-term memory, especially when we try to retain knowledge. The brain learns best in short bursts. It has been shown that twenty to forty minutes is the best amount of time for study; we retain most information then. Make notes during this time. After forty minutes, take a ten-minute break, then spend ten minutes trying to remember what you've learnt. Write it down and compare it with your notes. During the next few days, spend a few minutes going over the same information. The following week, reduce the review time to one or two minutes. This way you will fix what you have learnt in your long-term memory.

Oxygen is food for the brain

The brain accounts for only 2 per cent of our total weight, but it takes a quarter of the oxygen we inhale. When we use the brain by thinking, the flow of oxygenated blood to that particular part of it increases by 30 per cent. Conditions such as *arteriosclerosis,* when fat clogs up the arteries, causing the oxygen supply to the brain to diminish, seriously affect its ability to function. Many mental disorders in the older person can often be the result of a diminished oxygen supply to the brain, and are completely reversible.

Exercise stimulates the brain

Keeping physically active has a very positive effect on the brain. Not only does it increase your intake of oxygen but it also gives you a tremendous feeling of well-being. It has been found that people who exercise (a thirty-minute walk every day, for example) have better intellectual capacity, are more alert, are less depressed and have a better self-image than those who don't. Exercise also improves our balance, co-ordination, reaction times, and recognition memory, things that can dramatically deteriorate as we age.

Keep-fit classes where you exercise to music and have to remember steps and movements are great ways to stretch your brain. Sports such as tennis, golf, badminton and table tennis improve and maintain hand-eye co-ordination and are therefore excellent ways to keep fit and mentally alert.

Drinking and smoking can damage your brain

The long-term effects of chronic excessive drinking are well known. Though moderate alcohol consumption (a maximum of two units a day for women, three for men) is known to have certain health benefits, heavy drinking is harmful for both body and mind. The memory worsens dramatically after fifteen years of heavy drinking, or even sooner in people who go on binges.

The effects of long-term smoking on the brain are not as widely known. The carbon monoxide in each puff has a poisonous effect on the brain, and recent studies show that smokers have poorer memory than non-smokers as they age.

To keep your mind active you should

~ not smoke

~ keep your alcohol intake to a minimum

~ read a newspaper every day

~ do something that makes you think hard, such as doing a crossword or playing chess, draughts or Scrabble a few times a week

~ learn something new: go to language classes or learn a craft

~ change your routine regularly: do something different every week

~ improve your memory by making a mental image of names and numbers

~ memorise a poem or verse a few times a week

~ increase your oxygen intake by doing something physically active every day.

The Alzheimer's scare

Alzheimer's disease, first described in 1907 by Dr Alois Alzheimer, a German neurologist, is often mentioned in the context of ageing. It is a progressing condition of the brain, affecting memory, thought, and language. It is the most common form of *dementia*.

Alzheimer's disease affects one in twenty people over the age of sixty-five (most patients do not have any symptoms until around seventy-five). It touches all groups in society and is not linked with social class, sex, race, or geographical location. Though this disease has existed since ancient times, it seems to be increasing to an alarming degree. About 35,000 people in Ireland and 100,000 in Britain suffer from Alzheimer's disease.

The degenerative changes of Alzheimer's disease lead to patches or *plaques* in the brain and the entanglement of nerve fibres (*neurofibrillary tangles*), interfering with the interconnection between *neurons* (nerve cells in the brain). Memory loss and behavioural changes occur as a result of these changes in brain tissue. Alzheimer's is a slow, progressive illness. The early behavioural changes may not be noticed, especially difficulty with short-term memory; but as the disease progresses, memory loss increases, and there are changes in personality, mood, and behaviour. Lack of judgment, poor concentration, confusion and restlessness are all symptoms of Alzheimer's disease.

The disease silently destroys the brain. As the brain deteriorates, the rest of the body closes down, and patients can no longer care for themselves; they become dependent on others for help with all aspects of daily life. This care is usually provided by the family, lasting for many years. Patients normally die between two and twenty years after the appearance of the first symptoms.

The cause of Alzheimer's disease is unknown, and there is no cure. Ten per cent of Alzheimer's is of genetic origin, which often causes an early onset of symptoms, sometimes as young as thirty, though this is very rare.

Progress is being made in understanding the condition's basic biochemistry, and it is hoped that effective treatment will be available soon. Two drugs are available for treating Alzheimer's disease: *tacrine,* and *donepezil hydrochloride.* Both act to slow the breaking down of *acetylcholine* (a chemical necessary for the transmission of electrical signals between neurons) and so help communication between damaged brain cells. These drugs can slow down the rate of deterioration in some patients but cannot prevent death from the illness.

There are other types of dementia that can, in some cases, be successfully treated. It is important, therefore, to seek medical help if an older person shows symptoms of dementia to ascertain whether it is Alzheimer's. Only about half of all dementia is usually diagnosed as Alzheimer's disease.

The reason Alzheimer's disease appears to be on the increase is partly that it mostly affects people aged seventy-five to eighty and over, the fastest-growing population group in industrialised countries. It was quite rare for a patient to survive to that age in the past: the people who suffered from the disease would have died before they showed any symptoms. Medical science now manages to keep people alive much longer than before, which is why both the number of victims and the duration of the disease are increasing.

Alzheimer's disease is, of course, devastating for the sufferer, but it is also a great burden on the family. In the early stages, patients can be cared for in the home, but as the disease progresses this becomes increasingly difficult. Institutional care is inevitable at the later stages of the disease, which is largely paid for by the family of the sufferer. Few countries have a public health policy for patients with Alzheimer's disease. Most of the Alzheimer's associations, which provide information and support for families, are financed by charity.

Alzheimer's associations

Alzheimer's Society of Ireland

43 Northumberland Avenue

Dún Laoghaire

Co. Dublin

Phone: (01) 2846616

Western Alzheimer Foundation

Mount Street

Claremorris

Co. Mayo

Phone: (094) 62480

In Britain

Alzheimer Society

10 Greencoat Place

London SW1P 1PH

England

Phone: (0171) 3060606

Fax: (0171) 3060808

e-mail: info@alzheimer.org.uk

 ## Other forms of dementia

There are other diseases that have symptoms similar to those of Alzheimer's disease, such as *multi-infarct dementia* or stroke. A stroke is caused by problems with the circulation of blood to the brain. The brain needs a constant flow of oxygenated blood; if the flow is interrupted, parts of the brain die from lack of oxygen. This can be caused by a blood clot or a burst blood vessel.

You can have either a *major stroke,* which is sudden and very dramatic, even fatal, or a *minor stroke,* with milder symptoms, such as slurring of speech or numbness in a hand. A series of small strokes (*multi-infarct*) will cause loss of intellectual capacity, dementia to a greater or lesser degree, and some physical decline. Multi-infarct dementia accounts for between 12 and 20 per cent of all cases of dementia in people aged over sixty-five.

Senility

'Senility' is often mentioned when old people seem forgetful, repetitive, or clumsy. Even old people themselves talk about 'getting senile' when they seem to have lost some of their capacities.

What is senility? Is it a disease, or a condition that is inevitable? Can it be prevented?

The good news is that there is really no such disease, and it is not a condition that comes automatically with the ageing process. There are some changes in the way an older person thinks, but natural ageing does not include intellectual impairment, confusion, depression, or delusions. Those symptoms are due to disease and need to be diagnosed and treated. There are nearly a hundred disorders that mimic both dementia and Alzheimer's disease; all can be treated successfully.

Many people who are regarded as being senile are suffering from other problems, such as the wrong medication, depression, undetected hearing or sight problems, hypothermia, or alcohol abuse. Old people can easily become depressed, and this can be mistaken for dementia. Many cases of dementia can be cured, once the causes have been properly diagnosed.

 ## Conclusion

If you are in your sixties and can't remember where you put that piece of paper, or your second cousin's first name, should you worry that you are in the first stages of Alzheimer's disease? Of course not! Everybody's memory slowly deteriorates from the age of twenty. This is more noticeable after sixty, but that is normal. With a bit of luck and some stimulation of the brain, the chances are that your mind will remain alert until you die.

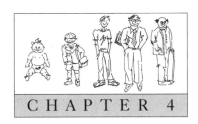

CHAPTER 4

FIT AFTER FIFTY
HOW TO KEEP FIT FOR LIFE

The human body was made to move—to walk, run, jump and climb, to pull and push and carry. This design was perfect for Stone Age people. Men and women needed to put their bodies through a lot of heavy work in order to survive.

Today we move very little in our daily lives. Work is less and less physically demanding, and our homes are full of labour-saving devices. Our body has not adapted itself to the modern passive life-style. Space Age humans have a Stone Age body.

We have to move our body every day to keep it healthy. As we age, exercise becomes even more essential. It is impossible to stay healthy in old age if we do not keep physically active. Unfortunately, older people tend to think they shouldn't move around too much, and often give up sports they previously enjoyed. This is a serious mistake. We need to maintain our heart, lungs, circulation, muscles and joints in good working order throughout life in order to prevent them from deteriorating.

 Dangers in your home

The sitting-room sofa is not good for our health, and the armchair is positively dangerous, because that is where we sit and, more often than not, have snacks while watching television. There is one type of chair that is a particular health hazard, and that is the reclining chair. This is a type of chair that reclines at the touch of a button, with a leg support coming out at the bottom. It makes the occupier half-lie as if in bed. Very comfortable! Some of these chairs also have a tilting mechanism that helps you get up, without using the muscles in your legs. (It is a very good device for a handicapped person, but most people who use these chairs are not handicapped.)

Some people love to spend hours in these chairs, watching television or reading. If, in addition, there is a kind friend or relative around who will bring you cups of tea and snacks, you may not have to move until it is time to go to bed. Many older people spend a large part of their day this way, thinking they don't have to move because they are old.

It's never too late to become active

But nobody is ever too old to move. A reasonably healthy person can take exercise at any age. While it's true that it's better to keep active all through life, it is possible for previously passive people to take up a physical activity and greatly improve their level of fitness and general health. Exercise is very beneficial in later life, and perfectly safe.

A number of research results illustrate the fact that the human body can stay fit and even grow stronger at any age. (See chapter 2.) We never lose the ability to improve our health. Loss of muscle mass in an older person is the result of disuse, not the inevitable result of advancing years. Many other signs of diminished physical capacity are also due more to a passive life-style than to age. Stiffness, lack of muscle strength and poor balance are often the cause of the falls that are so common among the elderly. Injuries from bad falls can be prevented by adopting a more active life-style, which should include muscle-strengthening activities. This will improve strength, flexibility, stamina, balance, and co-ordination, making us fit, strong, and able to be in charge of our own lives.

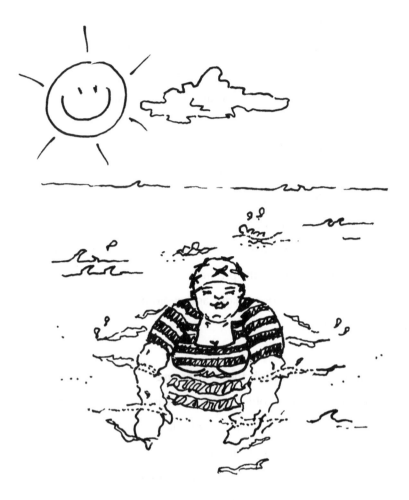

Why keeping active is essential

Physical activity—

~ reduces the risk of heart disease

Aerobic exercises—which include running, walking, swimming, cycling, and dancing—are all beneficial for the heart. They increase the demand for oxygen in the muscles, making the heart pump harder, thus increasing its strength little by little. Muscles that are made to work need oxygenated blood; this is supplied by the heart, which pumps the blood to the muscles. When we work the large muscle groups in our thighs and buttocks, the heart beats faster to meet the demand for energy. If we exercise regularly, our heart (which is itself a muscle) grows in strength and efficiency. In this way we also maintain good blood circulation through our entire body. That is why walking has to be included in your daily life. (You don't have to run, but you must walk.)

~ keeps weight under control

The well-known problem called 'middle-age spread' is due to a slower metabolism, an increasingly passive life-style, and an excessive intake of fat in our diet. As mentioned earlier, older people have the unfortunate tendency to adopt an increasingly passive life-style, and to overeat. This is why the majority of older people have a weight problem. If we make an effort to stay physically active, we can maintain our weight and avoid many conditions associated with being overweight.

~ prevents and manages high blood pressure

High blood pressure in an older person increases the risk of strokes and coronary heart disease. Obesity, smoking, high alcohol consumption and stress are among the factors that contribute to high blood pressure. It can also be hereditary. A combination of exercise and a low-fat diet can reduce high blood pressure and maintain it at a healthy level.

~ prevents bone loss

Our bone mass begins to decrease at about the age of thirty-five. *Osteoporosis*, a gradual and excessive thinning of the bones, affects mainly women but can also affect men. It is a hereditary condition but in women can be treated with *hormone replacement therapy.* A diet high in calcium, and regular weight-bearing exercise (running or walking), are advised for men. All older people, however, can maintain healthy bones with weight-bearing activities and a high intake of calcium.

~ **boosts energy levels**

Physical activity gives us more energy by increasing the circulation. Feeling tired is often due to the slowing down of the blood circulation that takes place when we are inactive. A brisk walk or any other exercise will often boost our energy level and stimulate our mind much more than taking a nap.

~ **helps manage stress**

It is a well-known fact that exercise greatly reduces stress. It makes us feel relaxed and helps us cope with all sorts of problems and hardships that life may bring. It also reduces depression.

~ **improves the quality of sleep**

Exercise makes us feel relaxed, even tired. This helps us fall asleep, and makes us sleep more deeply.

~ **makes us more independent**

A fit older person has no problem coping with the chores of daily life. Good muscle tone, co-ordination and balance make shopping, cleaning and even gardening a task that can be undertaken without too much effort. We do not have to rely on others to manage; this will give us a better self-image and improve our confidence.

In short, regular exercise is essential for quality of life as we grow older.

Keeping fit after fifty

If we keep active all through life, it will not be too hard to include physical activities in our daily life. The most important thing is to *move,* whatever activity we choose. But many older people settle into a comfortable, passive life-style that is hard to change. Once you get used to not doing very much it will seem difficult and tiring to do anything other than sit.

The modern world makes our lives more and more sedentary. Soon we will not even have to move to perform the simplest tasks. Shopping and banking can already be done on the internet; we send letters by e-mail; and most household chores are completed with little physical effort. In this way, the couch potato is well provided for. But we must make an effort to stay active, or our health will deteriorate at an alarming rate. If you enjoy organised activities, such as exercise classes or sports, you can keep up an exercise programme well into old age. Even if you have never exercised but you would like to try, it is possible to take up fitness classes or to learn such sports as tennis, badminton, or golf.

Some people hate exercise. In that case there are other ways of staying physically active and thus building up strength and stamina. Being fit means being strong and healthy, whether it is the result of organised sport or simply an active life-style.

If you like exercise

An ageing body needs exercise but, as I touched on earlier, of a different kind. We have to be aware of some limitations as we age. Our joints and back are growing more fragile. We have to treat our body with care if we want to stay mobile and therefore independent well into old age. But we must not go from high-impact aerobics to an armchair, from running or weight training to watching television. There are plenty of things in between.

The exercise routine that kept us fit in our twenties is not ideal for us as we grow older. We do need to move, but in a more gentle way. Older people need both more and less from their exercise routine. We need more of an immediate feeling of well-being, more enjoyment, variety, and information; we need less joint stress, strain, pain, and discomfort. When we were younger we exercised to burn fat, get fit, and look well. Now we want to exercise for vitality and mental alertness, to stay strong and independent.

But how can we know if the exercise routine we are starting is right for us? How do we know that it will not do more harm than good?

Here are some methods of choosing the right activity (and giving up the wrong ones):

~ **If it hurts, don't do it.** Don't do any movements that are painful or uncomfortable. If you have bad knees, avoid twisting or changing direction quickly. If you are over fifty, the same applies to your back. Treat it with care. Never bend forward and twist at the same time. Keep your knees slightly bent to save your back.

~ **If you are following a fitness class, make sure the instructor is experienced, and qualified to teach older people.**

~ **Change from high-impact (running and jumping) to low-impact activities.** Low-impact does not have to mean low-intensity, but it is more gentle on your joints, muscles, tendons, and ligaments. If you exercise to music, make sure the teacher uses music that is slow enough for you to be able to put your whole foot on the floor each time (from ball to heel). If you have to stay on your toes because the music is too fast, it may result in injury to your feet or ankles.

~ **Wear the right shoes.** Feet, ankles, shins, knees and backs are more vulnerable as we grow older. Protect them with shoes that support, stabilise and cushion your feet and also act as shock-absorbers. Buy good shoes for walking, tennis shoes for tennis, aerobic shoes for aerobics. In short, your shoes should suit the activity you intend to follow. Buy shoes in the afternoon, when your feet are bigger. Sports shoes should not have to be 'broken in': they should feel right the moment you put them on. If you can't afford new shoes, just make sure the ones you wear for walking are sturdy. Women should not walk in high heels.

~ **Drink plenty of water.** Our thirst mechanism does not work as well when we grow older. We need more water when we are exercising than when we are resting. Eight glasses of water a day is a good rule for an active person. During exercise, drink a few mouthfuls every ten minutes or so, and remember to keep drinking during the day.

~ **Train your muscles as well as your heart and lungs.** This benefits both bones and muscles. Use light weights, go to strength-training classes (of the kind that 'tone' your muscles), or do any activity that makes you pull, push, or lift. Gardening, DIY and housework are good examples of this. It will keep bones dense and muscles strong for life. Building muscle will also help you manage your weight, as toned muscles burn more energy.

~ **Ask your doctor.** If you are taking up any type of exercise for the first time, have a medical check-up to find out if you have any health problems to watch out for.

~ **Start any activity slowly.** Be patient with yourself in the beginning of a new activity. You don't have to exercise vigorously to see great benefits. Any amount of exercise will dramatically improve your health compared with a sedentary life-style. Exercise is a process. You have the rest of your life to perfect it.

A daily routine

The best way to make our lives more active is to incorporate exercise in our everyday routine, very much like the things we couldn't imagine not doing, such as brushing our teeth, or folding our clothes before going to bed. The three essential points to remember are: *like it, do it, make it a habit.* Find something you really like to do, that you would look forward to every day. Perhaps you would like to join a fitness, dancing or yoga class. If you are the gregarious type, ask a friend to join in, and make this the time that you get together. You may even be the kind of person who likes using exercise equipment in the home. There are so many machines on the market today, it is not hard to find something to suit you.

Stretching and warming up is very important before vigorous exercise. (This is not necessary when taking a walk.) It prepares your muscles, joints, heart and lungs for the work ahead. Cooling down slowly at the end of exercise should also be remembered.

When you have found an activity that you enjoy, look at your daily schedule, and find a time during the day when exercise is convenient and enjoyable. Decide whether the morning or the evening is your best time for exercise. If you are an 'early bird', it may suit you best to exercise in the morning. Many people find it easiest to do their physical activities before lunch; but it is just as beneficial at other times of the day.

The type of exercise you choose should suit your personality. If you like the company of others, a gym class or exercise to music may suit you. Or you may prefer to be alone and use this part of the day for thinking and unwinding. In that case, walking, running, swimming or using an exercise machine would be ideal. Some people like being supervised while exercising. Again, some sort of class is best in this case. The competitive person should play a game—tennis, badminton, or golf. Doubles tennis is fun and not very strenuous.

If your chosen activity is an outdoor one, it may sometimes be impossible to do it because of bad weather; so make sure you have some sort of indoor alternative. Swimming, badminton or exercise classes can all be enjoyed indoors. Exercise equipment at home can be used whatever the weather. If you vary your exercise routine regularly, you will not become bored and give up.

If you decide to buy exercise equipment to use at home, such as a stationary bike, treadmill, rowing machine, or weight machine, be sure beforehand that you will use it. Some people end up using these machines as clothes racks. Try out the machine if there are a few different brands of the same thing: there can be a huge difference in exercise bikes of different brands.

A good exercise routine might consist of three muscle-strengthening sessions a week, such as keep-fit, stretching, yoga or weight training, combined with three half-hour walks.

Don't overdo it! If walking for half an hour each day is comfortable, stick to that. If you want to increase the distance (and your fitness level), do so over time. Exercise for older people should be comfortable and enjoyable. If you overdo it, you may find it so strenuous that you give up.

If you don't like exercise

For some people, exercise is impossible—not because they are ill or disabled, but because any form of physical activity is totally alien to them. Some 'couch potatoes' are even proud of their inactive life and mock their more active friends. 'It's not my thing,' you often hear; 'I hate exercise,' or 'I get too tired.' If you are one of them and have never done anything more active than strolling to the end of the garden or lifted anything heavier than a loaf of bread, even light exercise will seem as impossible as climbing Mount Everest.

If you don't want to go to a keep-fit class—and a lot of older people do not—there are many ways to improve fitness that are easy and enjoyable. Recent studies also show that even light exercise benefits health. A daily walk of half an hour or more, combined with a little gardening or housework, is quite enough to give the average person a good level of fitness. All we need to do is think of an activity we enjoy, because that is the key to continued success. It's a bit like planning a meal: if you like it, you'll be back for more.

Nobody has the type of body that will stay healthy sitting around. So how can the person who hates exercise keep active? There are plenty of ways in which even the most ardent couch potato can move around and become fitter without doing that 'exercise thing' they hate and fear. Forget exercise: think 'doing' and 'moving'.

❯ Some tips for a more active life-style

Improve **aerobic fitness** (heart and lungs) by walking: ten minutes in the morning (walk to the paper shop), ten minutes at lunch time (walk around the garden or go to the grocer's to buy your lunch), ten minutes in the evening (walk the dog or take a stroll down the road to chat to a friend). Walk around the house during the commercial breaks on television. Or walk up a flight of stairs. If you live in a two-storey house, walk up and down the stairs ten times every day. It doesn't take too long and you don't have to go anywhere. (And don't tell anyone you're doing it if you don't want to ruin your 'couch potato' image.)

Get more **muscle strength** from lifting things. Lifting and carrying anything that is fairly heavy—groceries, laundry, books, small children—will make your muscles stronger. Housework is also a good way to work your muscles.

Become more **flexible** by reaching, bending, and twisting. Hanging up washing, putting books up on shelves, picking fruit or pruning bushes will stretch your muscles and ligaments, making them more supple, and increase blood circulation in those particular tissues.

Improve your **balance** by standing on one leg. Stand on one leg for a minute, then change legs. Poor balance is the main cause of injuries in falls, so common among the elderly. There are other ways to improve balance; try to think of some yourself.

What sitting still will do to your body

~ You will gradually put on more and more weight.

~ Your blood cholesterol level will increase.

~ Your blood pressure will rise.

~ You will risk developing heart disease.

~ The risk of having a stroke becomes higher.

~ Your immune system will be weaker and you will have less resistance to disease.

~ Your bones will become brittle.

~ Your energy level will decrease.

~ You will have poor muscle strength and flexibility, making it harder to perform everyday chores, which in turn will make you dependent on others.

~ You will not feel very well—and also, most probably, become grumpy.

If you are physically very passive, I'm sure this list of ailments will motivate you to get up from that chair and start to move around a bit more.

If you simply move around a little more every day it will improve your health very quickly. The results of recent medical studies show that even moderate exercise—

that is, simply moving our bodies a little every day—has a very beneficial effect on nearly every part of the body. It will lower both cholesterol levels and blood pressure, improve circulation, decrease body fat, and improve the immune system.

If you become a little more active, who knows? You may even like it! In any case, you will like the effect it has on the way you feel.

Ten tips to help you keep up physical activity

1. **Start now, and start slowly.** Once you have decided to become more active, make only one small change per day. If you are too ambitious in the beginning, you may become too tired and give up.

2. **Get the right fit.** Make sure your activity suits your schedule, life-style, and personality. Do something you enjoy and can fit into your day without too much disruption. (The best exercise is the one you'll do!)

3. **Get a dog.** The best way to force yourself to start walking is to own a dog. Dogs have to be exercised, and it is positively cruel to neglect this. Dogs are also lovely companions and bring a lot of pleasure. If you can't keep a dog, borrow somebody else's.

4. **Team up.** Get a friend to join you on your walks or exercise class. Friends often motivate each other to continue an activity.

5. **Inform yourself.** Learn about exercise and what works best for each part of the body. Ask a qualified fitness teacher for advice. Research has increased our understanding of exercise and its effect on the body; a fitness professional can advise you what activity is best for you. There are a lot of myths and methods in the popular press.

6. **Take a break.** If you don't feel like exercising, just do five minutes, promising yourself that you are allowed to stop when they are up. Once you are past the hurdle of the first few minutes, you probably won't want to stop.

7. **Be realistic.** Don't be upset if you don't experience a big difference in how you

feel at once. It takes time for your body to become used to a new routine. Be patient, and don't give up.

8. **Vary your routine.** Do a different type of exercise on alternate days to avoid boredom and injury. If all you do is walk, take a different route from time to time. If your activity is no longer a challenge, try something else. It will also stimulate your mind.

9. **Make exercise a treat.** Don't look at exercise as a treatment or medication. If you do something you enjoy, it will be a lot easier. Before long, you will look forward to your walk, game of tennis, swimming session, or yoga class; it will become the best part of your day. If you also perceive yourself as an active person you will have created a positive image of sport and exercise in your mind.

10. **Be proud of yourself.** Give yourself a pat on the back for any life-style change you make. Don't worry about missing a session: be proud of completed work-outs and the changes you have made in your life. Think of yourself as successful.

Conclusion

There's no getting away from the fact that the human body was made for movement. We have to move every day in order to stay healthy. Even though our ageing bodies can no longer perform at the same level as when we were younger, it is still possible to maintain an excellent level of fitness by taking exercise or just keeping physically active. It is not necessary to spend hours in the gym or to go to keep-fit classes every day in order to stay fit. The best methods of keeping fit are neither complicated nor expensive. If you simply take every opportunity to move your body during a normal day, you can raise your level of fitness very quickly. Try to find something you really like. It doesn't matter what you do, as long as you do it! Add some regular, moderate exercise, such as walking, and you will be very fit indeed.

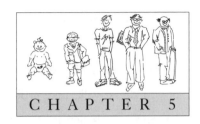

CHAPTER 5

STATE OF THE HEART
A HEALTHY HEART

Heart disease is the most common cause of death in the industrialised world. Up to ten years ago it killed twice as many men as women, but women are catching up fast, and heart disease is now the most common cause of death in the female population; five times as many women die of heart disease as of breast cancer.

Heart disease has reached almost epidemic proportions in the last ten years, and it is still increasing. Though it is mostly preventable, and we are bombarded with information on how to reduce the risks, most people pay little attention. It is as if we see heart disease as something that happens to other people, who 'catch' it or are born with a certain gene.

At least 65 per cent of all heart disease is caused by unhealthy living. The most common risk factors are smoking, high blood pressure, a high level of fats in the blood, and lack of exercise; other risk factors are obesity, stress, diabetes—and, yes, hereditary factors. Each one of these risk factors is bad enough on its own: two or more can be lethal. Combine smoking with a diet high in fat and lack of exercise, or a family history of heart disease with obesity and stress, and you have a recipe for disaster.

Blood, the heart, and blood vessels

The circulatory system of the average adult contains 4–5 litres of blood, which has four main constituents: *plasma,* which provides the liquid basis of the blood and contains sugar, urea, amino acids, mineral salts, and enzymes; *erythrocytes* (also called 'red blood cells'), which get their colour from *haemoglobin,* which carries oxygen and carbon dioxide; *leucocytes* (also called 'white blood cells'), whose function is to protect the body from infection (by increasing rapidly to kill the invasion of bacteria or viruses); and *platelets,* which are essential for the coagulation (clotting) of blood.

The heart is a muscle. It beats steadily in order to maintain the flow of blood through the body, day and night, all through life. Organs and tissues cannot survive without a constant supply of oxygen, nutrients, and warmth; waste products need to be taken away and expelled.

The heart takes care of every one of these needs. It consists of two pumps side by side. The blood makes two separate circuits, driven by these pumps, from and to the heart, known as the *systemic circulation* and the *pulmonary circulation.* In the systemic circulation, bright red blood containing oxygen is pumped from the left side of the heart into the main blood vessel in the body, the *aorta,* and then into a series of smaller arteries. These divide into smaller and smaller tubes, which finally become very fine hairlike vessels known as *capillaries,* which permeate the organs and tissues and supply them with oxygen and nutrients and also pick up waste products, such as carbon dioxide. These waste products are carried back to the heart by way of the *veins,* which join up to eventually form two large veins, the *superior vena cava* and *inferior vena cava,* before returning to the heart, this time to the right side, to be pumped through the lungs in what becomes the pulmonary circulation.

In the pulmonary circulation the oxygen-depleted blood—now slightly blue or purplish in colour—is pumped back into the lungs. Here the whole process starts again. The blood takes up a fresh supply of oxygen from the *alveoli,* the small air sacs in the lungs that contain the oxygen we inhale and expel the carbon dioxide that we exhale. The oxygenated blood then returns to the left side of the heart and again goes out into the body.

The ageing heart and blood vessels

As we grow older, our *cardiovascular* (heart and circulation) system becomes slower and less efficient, and there is a higher risk of something going wrong. The heart and blood vessels become steadily weaker, and the composition of our blood changes. The muscle cells of the heart degenerate, and the valves inside the heart, which control the direction of blood flow, thicken and become stiffer. As the built-in natural pacemaker that controls the heartbeat loses some of its cells, there may be a slightly slower heart rate.

The *electrocardiogram* (ECG) of a healthy older person is different from that of a younger adult. Abnormal rhythm (*arrhythmia*) is common in older people. There may also be a slight increase in the size of the heart. The heart wall thickens, which reduces the amount of blood the chamber can hold, and the heart fills more slowly.

The main artery from the heart, the aorta, becomes thicker and less elastic. This makes blood pressure higher, which in time makes the heart work harder. The other arteries also change in the same way. Most elderly people experience a moderate increase in blood pressure.

The body's natural receptors, which monitor blood pressure and help maintain an even pressure when we change position (for example from sitting to standing), become less sensitive with ageing. This results in a condition called *hypotension,* where blood pressure falls suddenly when you stand up, which may cause dizziness.

The walls of the capillaries thicken slightly, causing a slower exchange of nutrients and wastes.

The blood itself changes slightly with age. Ageing causes a reduction in total body water; as a result, there is less fluid in the bloodstream, which decreases the volume of the blood.

The number of red blood cells is reduced, which can contribute to fatigue. As the red blood cells are responsible for the supply of oxygen to organs and muscles, less oxygen means less energy. Most of the white blood cells remain the same, though certain cells important to immunity decrease in number, which can interfere with the ability to resist infections.

The effect of the ageing process

The heart of the average reasonably healthy older person continues to supply adequately all parts of the body with oxygenated blood. It will be slightly less able to tolerate increased work loads, because of a reduction in extra pumping ability (*reserve heart function*). Increased demands on the heart may result from illness, emotional stress, injury, extreme physical exertion, and some medication.

Coronary heart disease is not, however, an inevitable consequence of ageing. If we look after our health, our hearts should stay healthy as we grow older.

An unhealthy heart

Heart disease and its causes are complex. There is no single disorder that can be called 'heart disease': there are many different cardiac and circulatory disorders, with a range of causes involving either hereditary or environmental factors, or both. There may be a number of different causes for a single condition, each of them adding to the total picture and the resulting heart problem. The most serious condition, coronary heart disease, is usually attributable to many different factors.

❭ The most common disorders

The most common heart disorders in the older person are as follows.

Congenital heart disease is caused by malformations present from birth. Some of the deformities may be minor and can be missed unless specifically looked for. In the most crippling deformities, the 'used' (oxygen-depleted) blood bypasses the lungs and continues to circulate around the body. This causes the characteristic colour of the so-called 'blue baby'. Most heart defects can be corrected with surgery. Serious defects are extremely rare.

Atherosclerosis, or coronary artery disease, is the silting up of the arteries by deposits of fatty material called *atheroma.* The wall of the artery becomes partially clogged with deposits. A blood clot (*thrombosis*) may form on one of these deposits and lead to a complete blockage. The exact cause of the condition is not known, but various risk factors increase the chances of suffering from it: the most important are a family history of the condition, age, cigarette-smoking, a high-fat diet, high blood pressure, obesity, lack of exercise, and finally stress. It can affect any artery in the body.

Arteriosclerosis, on the other hand, is the hardening of the arterial wall brought about by degenerative changes, which increase with age. It is often confused with atherosclerosis, because of the similarity in many of the symptoms.

High blood pressure or *hypertension* is created when the force with which the blood flows is much greater than normal. It puts the whole circulatory system, including the heart and blood vessels, under great strain. High blood pressure that continues for many years can lead to several health problems.

Angina is not a disease in itself but a symptom of some underlying disorder, most commonly coronary heart disease. It is a tight, vicelike pain in the centre of the chest, often radiating to one or both arms, or the neck, which occurs when the heart is not receiving enough oxygen to meet an increased demand. This could happen during physical exertion or at times of extreme stress. The body becomes tense, and the blood pressure rises. At these times the heart temporarily needs more oxygen. A normal heart would have no problem with this demand; but when one or more of the coronary arteries (responsible for the blood supply to the heart) is narrowed, it interferes with the flow of oxygenated blood. The heart responds by producing the pain known as angina.

What is a heart attack?

A heart attack happens when there is damage to part of the heart muscle (the *myocardium*) because of a shortage of blood. This causes an interruption in the flow of blood around the body. A sudden reduction in the supply of blood to the heart can happen when one of the coronary arteries becomes blocked, either by a spasm or by a blood clot. The part of the heart that receives its supply of blood from the blocked artery can no longer work. If the spasm or blockage is relieved at once, the heart begins to function normally again. If, on the other hand, the blood supply is completely cut off, the cells change permanently within a few hours, and that part of the heart muscle is permanently destroyed. This is what is normally referred to as *infarct*.

A *myocardial infarction,* also called *coronary thrombosis* or *coronary occlusion,* is what is generally called a heart attack.

Sometimes the heart stops during a heart attack. Fatal *cardiac arrest* occurs in about half of all cases of heart attacks, usually before the victim can get medical attention.

 # Symptoms of heart disease

Heart disease can be difficult to diagnose, as the symptoms are as varied as the causes. Some people can have serious heart problems without any obvious signs.

Symptoms also differ between men and women. Under the age of fifty, men are three to five times more likely to die of heart disease than women. After the menopause, women have a greater risk, because of diminishing levels of *oestrogen,* a hormone that has a powerful protective effect on the heart by preventing atherosclerosis. By seventy-five, however, a woman's risk of developing heart disease is as high as that of a man. (Hormone replacement therapy can help lower the risks.)

Research shows that heart attacks in older women are more likely to be fatal, and women are also more prone to having a second heart attack. The reason may be that women have smaller hearts than men, and also smaller, narrower arteries.

Women do not always experience the same symptoms as men. In women the first signs of a heart attack may be a pain high in the abdomen, shortness of breath, and profuse sweating. There may simply be fatigue or a feeling of indigestion. Such rather vague symptoms can be wrongly diagnosed.

Women's heart problems also develop differently from those of men and often progress over a longer period. A woman may be more ill by the time she is seen by a doctor with suspected heart disease than a man who arrives at the casualty department with a heart attack. Women often have a wider variety of symptoms, which may cause doctors to explore causes other than a disorder of the heart.

How women and men differ in their symptoms

Women tend to experience chest pain as a tightness in the chest, radiating down the left arm or into the jaw. This can easily be mistaken for the pain of indigestion. Breathlessness as a symptom occurs more often in women. Fatigue associated with heart disease, which is usually overwhelming, also occurs more often in women. Dizziness, unexplained light-headedness, *oedema* (swelling) of the ankles or lower part of the legs, rapid heartbeat and nausea are symptoms common in a woman with a heart condition.

Men may feel a sudden pressure, fullness or squeezing pain in the centre of the chest that lasts more than a few minutes or is intermittent. They can also feel pain that radiates from the centre of the chest to the shoulders, neck, or arms. Chest discomfort accompanied by light-headedness, fainting, sweating, nausea or shortness of breath and a sudden onset of rapid heartbeats are also some of the common signs of heart problems in a man.

The risk factors

The main risk factors for heart disease are:

~ smoking

~ high blood pressure

~ high blood fat

~ obesity

~ lack of exercise

~ heredity

~ diabetes.

❱ Smoking

Everybody knows that smoking is bad for their health. If you still smoke despite the risks, you probably see the cigarette as a friend, rather than your worst enemy. I can only tell you what effect smoking has on your health. It's up to you to take the decision to stop.

Smoking affects the heart in many ways. Tobacco smoke contains about four thousand different chemicals, the most significant of which are nicotine and carbon monoxide.

Nicotine stimulates the production of stress hormones, which make the heart beat faster, causing a temporary rise in blood pressure, as well as an increase in the demand for oxygen. If the arteries are already affected by atherosclerosis, they will not be able to meet the demand.

Carbon monoxide is a poisonous gas, which causes oxygen deficiency in the blood. The arteries are damaged by this gas, which causes them to narrow and harden. Coagulation of the blood increases the danger of blood clots. These effects, taken together, greatly increase the risk of heart disease and thrombosis.

Smoking also causes lung cancer, *emphysema* (a disease that gradually destroys the lungs, making it difficult for the body to absorb oxygen), and other fatal illnesses.

❭ Myths about smoking

My grandfather smoked forty a day and lived until the age of ninety.

People who live to a great age despite an unhealthy life are freaks of nature and are the exceptions that prove the rule.

If you stop smoking you put on weight, which is just as dangerous.

It's true that smoking increases your *metabolism* (the rate at which the body burns calories). Many people also tend to eat more when they give up. But it is far more dangerous to smoke than to be overweight.

I've cut down on my consumption.

While cutting down on the number of cigarettes slightly reduces the risk to health, you are still damaging your heart and lungs. If you can successfully cut down on smoking, you can go one step further and stop. You will lose the smoker's cough, your breathing will improve, you will be fitter, and you will enjoy your food more. Isn't that worth the effort?

I've smoked for most of my life. It's too late to stop now.

It's never too late to stop smoking. The health risks resulting from smoking fall steadily, regardless of the age you are when you stop. The risks diminish particularly quickly during the first year after quitting; and after ten years your health will be close to that of a person who never smoked.

It's my business if I smoke: at least I'm not harming others.

Not true. There is now conclusive evidence that regular *passive smoking* (inhaling other people's smoke) is harmful. The spouse and children of smokers have a high incidence of chest infections and of certain cancers.

High blood pressure

As we saw earlier, the blood is pumped around the body by the heart, through the blood vessels, supplying all our organs with oxygen and nutrients. A certain pressure is needed for the blood to reach all parts of the body; the amount of pressure is decided by the contractions of the heart, by the kidneys, and by the smaller blood vessels. The faster the heart beats, and the more blood it pumps around the body, the higher the pressure.

The pressure is also affected by the amount of resistance the blood meets on its journey around the body. Blood pressure will increase if the blood vessels contract, or if there is a blockage.

Measuring blood pressure is a simple procedure that can be carried out by a doctor or a nurse. Most people will be familiar with the apparatus—a cuff made of fabric that is wrapped around the patient's arm and linked by a rubber tube to an inflation bulb.

Blood pressure is measured in two phases: *systolic pressure,* which is the pressure when the heart is contracted, and *diastolic pressure,* the pressure when the heart relaxes between beats. A pressure of 100–160 for systolic and 60–120 for diastolic is considered normal. Your result may be '140 over 90,' the higher number being systolic, the lower diastolic. An older person will often have a reading on the high side of normal.

Blood pressure can increase for many reasons, notably stress, physical exertion, drinking coffee or alcohol, smoking, or excess weight. About 5 per cent of patients have high blood pressure as a result of certain disorders, such as hormone imbalance or damaged kidneys. Some medicines can also cause an increase in blood pressure.

In the past, high blood pressure was thought to be an inevitable part of ageing. Recent studies among older people in Britain and the United States show, however, that blood pressure does not increase with age.

There are two ways to reduce blood pressure: a healthy life-style, and medication. A combination of the two is often the prescribed treatment.

Blood fats

Cholesterol, a fat-like substance that is used for many important functions, is found all through the body. But we must not have too much of it.

There is both good and bad cholesterol. 'Good' cholesterol (*high-density lipoprotein* or HDL) removes cholesterol from the blood by bringing it to the liver, where it is destroyed. 'Bad' cholesterol (*low-density lipoprotein* or LDL) contributes to the build-up of *plaque* in the arteries. Combined with other substances, plaque builds up on the walls of the arteries and can eventually cause a blockage. High cholesterol is mainly caused by too much animal fat in our diet, as well as a lack of dietary fibre, and also by too much sugar, alcohol, or coffee, by obesity, physical inactivity, and emotional stress.

The body also produces its own cholesterol; and in addition the level of fats in the blood is affected by how well our kidneys work.

The amount (and type) of fat in our diet is the most important factor influencing cholesterol levels, and also the most modifiable. A reduction in the intake of *saturated fat* (meat and dairy products) will dramatically reduce bad cholesterol. The fact that the inhabitants of certain countries, such as Italy, Greece, and Japan, have very low levels of cholesterol compared with people of northern Europe illustrates this point. It is well known that the so-called Mediterranean diet is beneficial for the heart and circulation, and healthier than diets in northern Europe.

I describe a healthy diet in detail in chapter 6; but there is one product that is particularly beneficial for the heart that I will mention here. Benecol, a butter substitute, has recently been introduced on the Irish and British market. Not only does it keep your cholesterol level down, it actually reduces it. Benecol has been used in Finland since 1995 and has been proved to greatly improve the health of patients with high cholesterol, thus reducing the risk of heart disease. It is believed that 20 grams of Benecol a day will block 'bad' cholesterol from being absorbed into your bloodstream and will maintain 'good' cholesterol levels. Of course it does not mean that you can indulge in unhealthy foods, expecting Benecol to act as an antidote: you still have to keep animal fats to a minimum, and try not to put on too much weight.

Excess weight

Your heart has to work harder the more weight you carry. Your blood pressure will increase and your arteries may harden, which increases the risk of heart disease.

Where the extra fat is situated makes a big difference. If you store excess fat around your waist and chest, the risk is greater. The fat cells that are stored in the abdominal cavity and around the intestine are more easily activated by stress hormones than those stored on hips and thighs. The fat can also get into the bloodstream and end up stored in the walls of the arteries, which can cause blood clots. Excess fat in women is usually stored on hips, buttocks, and thighs, which is not as dangerous for the heart.

Lack of exercise

As regular exercise improves the circulation and protects the heart, a sedentary life-style is one of the most important risk factors for heart disease. Exercise makes the heart muscle strong and helps you cope with physical strain. Your blood pressure becomes lower, your blood circulation is improved, and your body is able to take in more oxygen. In addition, physical activity reduces the risk of blood clots. Regular exercise will also help maintain your weight within healthy levels, help you cope better with stress, and improve your mood.

Hereditary factors

Even though heart disease is largely preventable, it is, in some cases, inherited. If you come from a family where heart disease has struck several members (parents, grandparents, brothers or sisters), your risk is higher than if there has been no heart disease in your family. It is not certain how the tendency for heart disease is inherited. Some of the risk factors, such as high blood pressure and extremely high levels of blood cholesterol, are partly inherited. It is up to the individual to be aware of a family history of heart disease. Mention this to your doctor, have regular check-ups, and try to adopt a healthy life-style.

 ## Diabetes

The *pancreas* (a gland situated below the kidneys) secretes a hormone called *insulin,* which regulates the level of sugar in the blood and the conversion of sugar into heat and energy. If you do not have enough insulin, it will result in the disease known as diabetes, which exists in two forms: *juvenile diabetes,* an inherited condition occurring in children and young adults, and *maturity-onset diabetes,* a less severe form affecting people over twenty-five. Sufferers from this kind of diabetes tend to have high cholesterol levels, to be obese, and to suffer from high blood pressure.

Juvenile diabetes is usually treated with daily insulin injections. Maturity-onset diabetes is less severe and is normally controlled by a low-carbohydrate diet combined with sugar-reducing drugs.

❭ Alcohol and the heart

The good news is that light to moderate consumption of alcohol reduces the risk of heart disease. Alcohol in small quantities raises the levels of 'good' cholesterol in the blood. But it is only beneficial if taken in moderation: over-indulgence can raise blood pressure, increase 'bad' cholesterol levels, and cause excess weight.

A moderate level of alcohol means 21 units per week for a man and 14 for a woman (a 'unit' meaning a helping, i.e. a glass of wine or beer, a shot of whiskey or brandy). These limits vary slightly from one medical study to another, but it is important to try to keep alcohol consumption at around those levels.

 ## Stress

Our ancestors led a hard and dangerous life. They had to be able to both fight and run away from wild animals. Their bodies were designed to cope with this kind of life; and so are ours.

When we are under stress, the *adrenal glands,* situated on top of the kidneys, produce a hormone called *adrenalin,* which raises both blood pressure and blood sugar and makes the heart beat faster. It makes us ready to respond quickly to fear or anger. Stress helps the body respond to a threat, real or imagined; this is what is known as the 'fight or flight' response.

If you can respond to stress in a physical way, it is much better for your heart; it is the fact that we usually have to suppress the need to run or fight that can damage the heart. A certain amount of stress is necessary in our life. It is stimulating and challenging; it makes life interesting and fun. But too much of it is harmful.

If there is too much stress in our daily life, the effects can become chronic. The raised blood pressure, faster heartbeat and raised blood sugar levels will be permanent and will cause other disorders. A person suffering from stress may have chest discomfort, breathlessness, palpitations, tension headaches, tiredness, indigestion, diarrhoea, frequent urination, even high blood pressure.

Many things in our life can cause stress, such as the death of a close family member, divorce, loss of a job, taking out a mortgage, problems at work, and many others. How we cope with stress is very individual: what may cause one person terrible distress may not be so terrible for another. It also depends on our general health and our personality. Talking about our problems to a friend or relative can be a great help. Exercise, enough sleep, taking time off for hobbies or to meet friends, learning relaxation methods, massage, reading and listening to music are some ways of reducing stress. Trying to reduce your work load, and perhaps learning to say 'no' to demands for extra work, could also help. In other words, take it easy! It will make you feel a lot better.

Panic: the heart attack that isn't

A *panic attack* is often mistaken for a heart attack. In fact it has nothing to do with heart disease.

A panic attack is caused by severe anxiety, which makes the body respond by going on alert, reacting as if you are faced with an immediate threat from an enemy. This is a mechanism that was useful for Stone Age people, who often needed an immense surge of energy when faced with danger. Severe stress floods the body with adrenalin, triggering a release of energy. Muscles tense, and heartbeat and breathing become more rapid, which is useful if you need to run fast from danger; but if the threat is in the mind, there is nowhere to run.

The symptoms of a panic attack can be so frightening that you end up going to hospital, only to be told that you are 'merely' suffering from stress. Panic attacks can cause symptoms such as heart palpitations, dizziness, fainting, shortness of breath, nausea, shaking, numbness in fingers and toes, and sweating. Some people can even feel as if they are dying.

Panic attacks have become more common than ever before, perhaps because of the increased pressure of modern living. Five per cent of the population of Britain suffer from panic attacks at some stage in their lives. Women are more prone to it than men.

There are different ways of treating *panic disorder* (repeated panic attacks). Some drugs, such as Valium, are known to help in certain cases, as well as other antidepressants. *Breath therapy* (teaching sufferers to breathe more slowly), counselling and relaxation methods can also be useful.

Eight ways to a healthier heart

1. Don't smoke.

2. Take regular exercise.

3. Reduce animal fat in your diet.

4. Include cholesterol-reducing foods in your diet.

5. Keep your weight down.

6. Reduce stress by relaxing and taking time off.

7. Have regular medical check-ups (once a year), controlling blood pressure, cholesterol levels, and weight.

8. Be careful with your alcohol intake: stay within recommended limits

 # Conclusion

Apart from hereditary factors and diabetes, it is possible to reduce most of the risk factors of heart disease. Changes in life-style are difficult to achieve, demanding determination, self-discipline, and hard work. But if you really want to keep your heart healthy and as a result feel well, you will succeed. Do not wait for inspiration to suddenly hit you. It won't. Decide now, draw up a plan, and follow it.

It is important, however, not to do too much at once. Take it one step at a time, and adjust slowly to a new life-style. Set goals that are realistic. If you are too ambitious, the chances are that you will be disappointed and give up if you don't reach your goal at once. Your brain is better at receiving positive messages than negative ones. Say, 'I will eat more fruit and vegetables,' rather than 'I must not eat cakes and biscuits'; or 'I will walk for half an hour a day,' not 'I won't watch television all afternoon.' Be proud of any changes for the better. Believe in yourself, and enjoy the feeling of improved health.

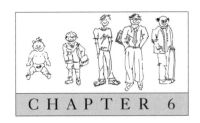

CHAPTER 6

THE PROOF OF THE PUDDING
THE OLDER PERSON'S HEALTHY DIET

Food is the fuel for the human body: we need to eat for energy, growth, body function, and tissue repair. We require certain nutrients to stay healthy. But food is much more than that: it is probably the most important thing in life. Eating is associated with our emotions, memories, and feelings of pleasure. We gather around a meal with our family each day, and the most important moments in life are usually celebrated with a dinner. Our earliest memories are connected with food; our eating habits, our likes and dislikes are often created in early childhood.

If hunger was the only reason for eating, a healthy diet would be easy to achieve. But because certain foods contain chemicals that make us feel happy, and other foods awaken pleasurable memories, we often want to eat things that are bad for our health in quantities that exceed the recommended amounts. As a result, we often endanger our health by our eating habits.

Traditional dishes

Most countries have traditional dishes, which often consist of the food that was available to people centuries ago. That is why diet in northern Europe is so different from that of countries further south. In the past, fruit and vegetables were not easy to come by in the north, and the diet in those countries was often high in animal fats and low in fruit and vegetables. Countries around the Mediterranean had, and indeed still have, a very healthy diet, rich in carbohydrates, fruit, vegetables, olive oil, and fish. This type of diet has spread further north and is now becoming more popular everywhere. Italian and Greek cuisine can be found in most countries today, which is a good thing. A meal of pasta with tomato sauce, or grilled fish with vegetables cooked in olive oil, is far healthier than steak and chips.

Unfortunately, we are still attached to food that we associate with our countries' traditions and often eat meals that will increase our cholesterol level and make us put on weight. It is very difficult to persuade a Scandinavian to give up his meatballs with gravy, a Belgian his chips and mayonnaise, an Englishman his roast beef and Yorkshire pudding. A German would not find it easy to live without sausages, and an Irishman would be heartbroken at the thought of going without bacon, eggs, sausages, and black pudding.

Eaten only occasionally, this type of food will not do too much damage. We can still enjoy traditional foods on special occasions, provided our daily eating habits are reasonably healthy.

 ## A healthy diet

We need to eat food that contains all the nutrients for the body to undertake all its functions. The human body needs carbohydrates, fats, protein, vitamins and minerals in certain quantities every day, all through life. Diets low in fats and high in carbohydrate, dietary fibre, fruit and vegetables are the healthiest.

❭ Carbohydrates

Carbohydrates are the body's greatest source of energy. They are divided into two types: sugars and starches.

The most common **sugars** are *glucose, fructose,* and *galactose.* Sugar added to food and drink, as well as soft drinks and sweets, is the principal source in our diet. Sugar is also added to some processed foods, such as soup, tinned fruit and vegetables, baked beans, and some meat products. In Ireland and Britain the average diet contains between 14 and 26 per cent sugar, which provides only calories and contains no other nutrients. Too much sugar in your diet will result in tooth decay and vitamin and mineral deficiencies.

Starches, or complex carbohydrates, are found in plant food. Starches from vegetables, pulses, seeds and fruit provide a slow-release energy over a longer period. This prevents drastic swings in blood sugar levels and gives us sustained energy. *Unrefined starches,* such as whole-grain bread, pasta, rice, beans, and potatoes, are the best type of carbohydrate. Apart from energy, they provide the body with certain proteins and many vitamins and minerals. They are also a very good source of fibre.

All carbohydrates provide energy. Sugar increases the level of insulin in the blood, which rapidly converts it into heat and energy. This energy depletes very quickly and results in feelings of fatigue.

❭ Fibre

Medical research has proved that a high intake of complex carbohydrates can help reduce the risk of heart disease and bowel cancer. Dietary fibre, found in these foods, is an essential part of a healthy diet, even though it contains no nutrients. It consists of plant cellulose and other indigestible material, such as pectin and gums. Fruit, vegetables, whole-grain bread, nuts and pulses are all good sources of dietary fibre.

The chewing of fibre stimulates the flow of saliva, adding bulk and helping with the digestion and absorption of nutrients. *Pectin,* a soluble fibre found in apples and carrots, encourages the elimination of waste products from the blood and helps balance blood sugar levels. Fibre also helps control the body's cholesterol level. If your diet contains enough fibre, any excess cholesterol is excreted with all the other waste materials.

❭ Protein

Protein is responsible for maintaining the structure of the body. About 20 per cent of the human body is made of protein, including muscles, bones, skin, nails, and hair.

Protein is made of twenty-three different *amino acids,* of which the body can produce fifteen. We have to obtain eight other amino acids from proteins in our diet: these are called *essential amino acids* and are found in meat, fish, eggs, dairy products, and certain fruit and vegetables.

Most diets in the West contain sufficient amounts of protein—indeed most people eat a lot more than they need. A lack of protein in the diet can retard growth

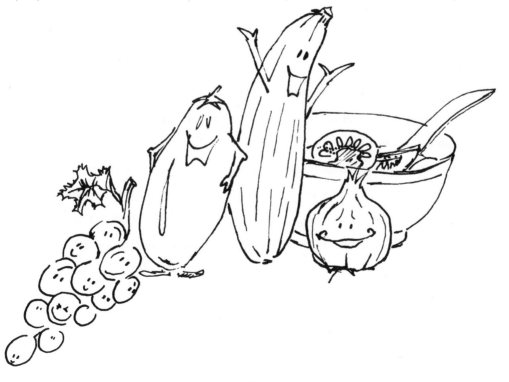

in children and cause fatigue in adults; too much protein can put a strain on the liver and kidneys and increase the risk of certain cancers and even heart disease.

It is better to get the protein we need from non-animal sources. All unrefined food contains a lot of protein, such as rice (8 per cent), potatoes (10 per cent), oranges (8 per cent), and beans (26 per cent).

About 15 per cent of our daily calorie intake should come from protein. The average adult needs only 60 grams (2 oz) of protein a day, which is the equivalent of a small piece of meat or chicken.

Fats

Fats are an important source of energy, particularly for the nervous system. They also contain vitamins A and D. Fat is stored in the body in special cells that form pads of tissue under the skin, which are used to protect vital organs, to protect us from shock, and to insulate us from cold. The body stores excess fat, which can be used for energy if there is a shortage of food. A man with 15 kg (33 lb) of stored fat could support life for two months. Obese people can have up to 100 kg (220 lb) of fat on their body, which is equivalent to a year's supply.

Fats are found in meat, fish, dairy products, and vegetable oils. A certain amount of fat in our diet is essential for good health, and a completely fat-free diet could be dangerous. The problem with fat, however, is that we tend to eat too much, and the wrong kind.

Too much *saturated (animal) fat* in our diet can seriously damage our health. It causes high cholesterol, heart disease, cancer, strokes, and obesity. Saturated fat clogs the arteries, adds extra weight, and prevents the absorption of nutrients.

While vegetable oils are much better for us, they can cause problems if they are *hydrogenated,* which means the oil has been processed to change it from liquid to solid in order to use it in processed foods. Oils solidified in this way turn into saturated fats, with the same dangers as animal fats. Look for the word 'hydrogenated' on the label of foods you buy, and try to eliminate them from your diet.

The good fats are *mono-unsaturated* and *polyunsaturated* fats. Mono-unsaturated fats are found in olive, canola (rape seed), sesame seed, peanut and walnut oil. Polyunsaturated oils are found in fish, nuts, and seeds. These fats have a protective effect on the heart, and will even lower cholesterol.

All fats, good or bad, contain the same amount of calories, however, and too much will result in weight gain, which in turn can damage your health. Fat has twice the calories of the other main nutrients, protein and carbohydrate. To make your diet more healthy, try to cut down on your intake of fats, and use small amounts of good fats instead of animal fats.

How to cut down on fat

~ Use olive oil instead of lard or butter when cooking, and keep the amount to a minimum.

~ Use pure vegetable-oil spreads (such as Flora or Benecol) instead of butter or margarine made with hydrogenated oil.

~ Grill, boil, bake or stir-fry instead of frying.

~ Cut down on high-fat dairy products, such as cream and cheese, and change to skim milk, low-fat yoghurts, and low-fat cheese.

~ Eat fatty fish (salmon, sardines, mackerel, herring, or trout) at least once a week.

Vitamins

Vitamins are compounds found in certain foods that the body needs for growth, function, energy, tissue repair, and waste removal. They are divided into water-soluble and fat-soluble vitamins.

Water-soluble vitamins (vitamins B and C) have to be included in our daily diet, as they are not stored in the body, and any excess is excreted in the urine.

A *recommended daily allowance* (RDA) for vitamins has been established by international health organisations. This is the level of nutrients believed to meet the needs of the average adult. It is sometimes given in terms of the *international unit* or *IU.* (The IU number is usually printed on the label.)

There are seven types of **vitamin B**. *Thiamine* (also known as vitamin B_1) is responsible for converting blood sugar into energy, promoting growth, and keeping the nervous system healthy. It is found in all plant and animal food, such as whole-grain products, brown rice, seafood, and beans. RDA: 1 mg.

Riboflavin (also known as vitamin B_2) is good for cells, growth, and reproduction, and is essential for the body in producing energy. Vitamin B_2 is found in milk and dairy products, green leafy vegetables, liver, kidneys, and yeast. RDA: 1.3 mg.

Niacin (also known as vitamin B_3) is essential for the production of sex hormones, for energy, the nervous system, and the digestion. Meat, fish and poultry, peanuts and avocados are good sources. RDA: 18 mg.

Panothenic acid (also known as vitamin B_5) helps us fight infections, heal wounds, strengthen the immune system, and build cells. It is found in liver, kidneys, fish, eggs, chicken, nuts, and whole-grain products. RDA: 7 mg.

Pyridoxine (also known as vitamin B_6) is found in meat, eggs, whole-grains, yeast, cabbage, melon, and molasses. Its function is to aid the nervous system and the production of cells. It is important for a healthy immune system and for maintaining leucocytes (white blood cells), which produce antibodies. RDA: 1.5 mg.

Cyanocobalamin (also known as vitamin B_{12}) is obtained by eating fish, dairy products, beef, pork, lamb, offal, eggs, and milk. It helps us produce erythrocytes (red blood cells), increase energy, improve memory and concentration, and maintain the nervous system. It also promotes growth in children.

Folic acid (also known as vitamin B_c) is found in leafy green vegetables, yeast, liver, carrots, avocados, and apricots. Folic acid is vital for the red blood cells (for carrying oxygen) and for the metabolism of sugar. It also protects against foetal abnormalities. RDA: 200 µg (micrograms).

Vitamin B is very important for most of the body's functioning. Ensuring that you take in enough every day may seem very complicated; but if you study the list above you will see that most of the different vitamin Bs are found in the same foods; if your diet includes a little of each food group you will receive adequate amounts for all your body's needs each day. Eat some whole-wheat bread, milk, green vegetables, meat or fish every day and an egg a few times a week and you will get plenty of vitamin B.

The second water-soluble vitamin is **vitamin C** (also called *ascorbic acid*). It is found in fresh fruit, berries, vegetables, and potatoes. Vitamin C is essential for healthy skin, bones, and muscles, for healing, protection from viruses and allergies, and good vision. It also lowers the level of cholesterol and aids the absorption of iron. It is very important to have vitamin C in your daily diet. If you eat some fruit (for example an orange and an apple) every day you will cover your vitamin C needs. RDA: 40 mg.

Fat-soluble vitamins (vitamins A, D, E, and K) are absorbed by the intestine and carried to the different parts of the body by the *lymphatic system,* which is part of the immune system. Fat-soluble vitamins are important, as they are responsible for maintaining the structure of our cells.

Vitamin A is found in liver, kidneys, eggs, butter, fish oils, and the *beta-carotene* of dark-green and yellow fruit and vegetables. As vitamin A is fat-soluble, it is a good idea to put a small amount of fat (preferably olive oil) on cooked vegetables to help the body absorb it more efficiently. It is needed for strong bones, good vision, and healthy skin; it also improves the body's ability to heal. RDA: 700 µg. Too much vitamin A is harmful, especially during pregnancy.

Vitamin D can be found in milk products, eggs, fatty fish, and fish oil, and is absorbed by the skin from sunlight. It is important for growth, strong bones and teeth and helps in the absorption of calcium. RDA: 800 IU for people over sixty-five.

Vitamin E, which you can find in nuts, seeds, eggs, milk, whole-grain, leafy vegetables, avocados, and soya, is necessary for the absorption of iron, the protection of the circulation, the slowing of the ageing process, and fertility. RDA: not yet established.

Vitamin K, obtained from green vegetables, milk products, apricots, whole-grains, and cod-liver oil, helps the clotting of blood and helps heal wounds.

❭ Minerals

Minerals are metals that work in a similar way to vitamins and in addition provide the structure for teeth and bones. Minerals exist in two groups: *major minerals,* which are those that are needed in quantities of more than 100 mg per day, and *trace elements,* of which only small amounts are required.

The **major minerals** are calcium, iodine, iron, chromium, magnesium, and potassium.

Calcium, which can be found in dairy products, leafy green vegetables, broccoli, and tofu (soya-bean curd), is necessary for the production of hormones, for maintaining strong bones, for the muscles, nervous system, and blood pressure, and for metabolising iron. RDA: varies according to age, but the minimum for young adults is 700 mg, for those over forty, 1,200 mg.

Iodine, from fish and seafood, pineapples, raisins, seaweed, and dairy products, helps produce hormones from the thyroid gland and is also good for healthy hair, skin, and teeth. RDA: 140 µg.

Iron is one of the most important minerals, because it ensures that the blood is able to carry oxygen. It is found in liver, kidneys, red meat, pulses, broccoli and other dark-green vegetables, nuts, and egg yolks. RDA: 18 mg for women, 9 mg for men.

Chromium is a mineral mainly present in liver, whole-grain cereals, meat, and cheese, and it is responsible for stimulating the production of insulin. RDA: 25 µg.

Magnesium, found in brown rice, soya beans, nuts, whole-grains, dark chocolate, and legumes, is needed by the body for the repair and maintenance of cells and most other processes, such as nerve impulses and the growth and repair of bones. RDA: 300 mg.

Potassium, from avocados, leafy green vegetables, bananas, dried fruit, vegetable and fruit juices, potatoes, nuts, and molasses, is needed for leucocytes (red blood cells) and for nerve and muscle functions. RDA: not applicable.

These are the most important vitamins and minerals. If you include the major food groups in your diet—carbohydrates (bread, potatoes, rice, pasta), protein (meat, fish, eggs, dairy products, certain fruit and vegetables), and fats—you will certainly meet your body's vitamin and mineral needs.

A vitamin and mineral supplement in the form of a daily tablet is also a good idea, because it will ensure that any imbalance in your diet is corrected before it causes health problems. It is unwise, however, to take too much of any one vitamin, as it could have a harmful effect. The only exception to this rule is vitamin C, which, if you have a viral infection, can be taken in very high doses for a short period. As vitamin C is water-soluble, any excess is excreted in the urine.

⟩ Salt

Most people eat too much salt, which, if taken in excess, is believed to cause high blood pressure, water retention, and kidney and heart problems. Ideally we should eat only 5 g of salt a day, which is about half the amount in the average diet. Most of the salt we eat has already been added to manufactured food, such as crisps, soup, cereal, bread, cheese, bacon, ham, smoked fish and meat, and soda water.

If you try not to add salt to your meals, using herbs and spices instead, you could halve your salt intake.

That middle-age spread

The older we are, the more difficult it is to keep slim. This is not because of hormones or hereditary factors but because of the slowing down of our *metabolic rate* (the rate at which our body burns energy). Older people also tend to eat more and to exercise less. The pleasures of the table and less enthusiasm for physical activity, combined with a slower metabolism, contribute to a thickening waistline in older people. But if we try to cut down on fat in our diet and try to move around a bit more, we can stay reasonably slim as we age.

The older person's diet

A healthy diet is essential as we grow older. Many ailments that afflict older people are indirectly caused, or at least worsened, by an inadequate intake of essential nutrients, dietary fibre, and water. Conditions such as heart disease, osteoporosis, diabetes, kidney disease and even cancer are influenced by our diet.

Studies show that old people generally do not make an effort to make their diet healthy, whether they are rich or poor. This may be because of a lack of information or an unwillingness to change eating habits for the better. Older people's dietary requirements differ from those of younger adults: certain vitamins and minerals are more important as we grow older and our bodies change.

Older people have a poorer thirst mechanism. It is important, therefore, to remember to drink eight glasses of water a day to keep the body hydrated. Without enough water, blood pressure may fall dangerously low, blood clots may form, blood vessels and kidney function can be badly affected, and there may be a risk of constipation.

It is also important to consume more grain-based foods, such as bread, cereal, rice, and pasta, as well as fruit, vegetables, and low-fat dairy products, and less meat, fats, oils, and sweets.

It has been found that older people do not get enough calcium, vitamin B_{12} or vitamin D from their diet, and many need to take vitamin supplements to cover their needs for these essential nutrients.

❭ Why we can't do without calcium

Calcium is important for keeping bones strong. It has recently been discovered, however, that calcium plays a much wider role in the body's structure and health. It has an influence on every major organ in the human body.

Calcium does indeed keep bones strong. But bones are not the final destination of calcium—they are in fact the starting point. Bones continuously release calcium into the body, where it plays a central role in controlling blood pressure and in women easing menstrual problems. It is also required for many other bodily functions, such as the transmission of nerve impulses that control muscle contractions, the release of chemicals that carry messages between nerves, and binding together cells to form organs. Calcium is also responsible for the regulation of digestion, the metabolism of fat, the release of energy, the production of saliva, the clotting of blood, the secretion of hormones, and growth. Recent research suggests that calcium may protect us from cancer of the breast, prostate gland, and pancreas.

If we don't take in enough calcium in our diet, the *parathyroid hormone* (secreted by the parathyroid gland behind the thyroid gland in the neck) signals the release of the mineral from the bones. That is how bone depletion starts, and that is also why we have to make sure we get enough calcium every day as we age. For an older person, 1,200 mg of calcium a day is the minimum required. Three glasses of low-fat milk and a helping of calcium-rich vegetable (broccoli, cabbage, or spinach) will cover your daily needs.

Vitamin D

This vitamin is also essential for older people. It plays an important part in helping our body maintain proper levels of calcium and is important for the immune system. It is vital for the health of our skeleton. In children, a lack of vitamin D can lead to rickets, and in older people it can cause osteoporosis.

Vitamin D is mainly *synthesised* or produced in the skin in response to sunlight. If we don't get enough through sunlight, we have to make sure we get it in our diet. Recent warnings about the danger of skin cancer from sunlight have resulted in vitamin D deficiency in young women. Older people, especially those who are housebound, also run the risk of not getting enough vitamin D.

The recommended daily allowance of vitamin D is 400 IU for young adults and 800 IU for people over sixty-five. Fifteen minutes of sunlight on your skin per day is enough and will not cause an increased risk of skin cancer. In winter, especially in northern Europe, vitamin D supplements in the form of cod-liver oil capsules are recommended.

Antioxidants and cancer

Nutrients called *antioxidants,* such as vitamin C, vitamin E, beta-carotene and the minerals zinc and selenium, found in fruit, vegetables, and nuts, are known to have an anti-ageing effect. They are also the body's protection against the *free radicals,* which cause cancer. Vitamins C and E have long been known to be powerful antioxidants, and recent research shows that vitamin A, selenium, zinc and copper also have the same qualities.

The American Cancer Society estimates that diet is a primary factor in a third of all cancers. This conclusion has been derived from thousands of studies of people throughout the world, and it is supported by findings in laboratory cell cultures and experimental animals. These studies suggest that a change in eating habits, increasing the consumption of fruit and vegetables and eating less red meat and saturated fats can significantly reduce the risk of developing most of the common cancers, such as colon, lung, bladder, stomach, oesophagus, mouth, throat and breast cancer.

There is no guarantee, of course, that adopting a particular diet can ensure that you won't get cancer. But the evidence strongly suggest that eating a lot of fruit and vegetables does protect the body from free radicals.

An apple a day

A daily intake of at least three helpings of fruit is an important ingredient of a healthy diet. The easiest way to eat a variety of fruit is to make fruit salad. Make up a bowl of different fruit chopped into small pieces—an orange, an apple, a banana, some kiwi fruit, a pear, and some grapes. Sprinkle it with unsweetened orange juice, keep it in the fridge, and have at least two helpings a day. It is delicious and filling; it may even help you cut out sugary and fatty snacks.

Eating for a healthy heart

Reducing fat in our diet is known to be beneficial for the heart. But that is only half the picture. It is not the amount of fat that matters but, as we have seen, the kind of fat.

Saturated fats are the culprits when it comes to high cholesterol and blocked arteries, and they have to be kept to a minimum. They are found in chicken fat (mainly in the skin), vegetable shortening (hydrogenated vegetable oil), lard, beef fat, and butter.

Recent studies indicate that reducing total dietary fat is less effective in reducing cholesterol than replacing saturated fats with unsaturated fats. One study showed that every 5 per cent increase in saturated fat in the diet resulted in a 17 per cent increase in the risk of cardiovascular disease.

Fats that are good for the heart include those found in fish, olives, avocados, seeds, and nuts. For cooking and salad dressing choose from olive, sesame seed, peanut and walnut oils. Be sure to use them sparingly: even 'good' oils are high in calories, and putting on weight will increase the risk of high cholesterol and heart disease.

Other foods that are good for the heart include fish (at least once a week), soya protein, whole-grain food (brown bread and rice), calcium (either from food or supplements), tea (a rich source of *flavonoids,* protective antioxidants), and a moderate consumption of alcohol (one drink a day for women, two for men).

Ten things you should eat to age better

Recent research has proved that the following food items can help slow down the ageing process:

1. **Tomatoes** contain a strong antioxidant, called *lycopene,* which reduces the risk of cancer and increase survival for cancer patients. It also improves mental function in old age and decreases the risk of heart disease. There is more lycopene in tomato sauce and in cooked and canned tomatoes than in fresh tomatoes.

2. **Olive oil** is the main component of Mediterranean diets and has been proved to reduce death from disease and cancer. Olive oil also contains antioxidants.

3. **Purple grape juice and wine** have significantly more antioxidants than orange juice and tomato juice. Research has shown that drinking red wine in moderation (one or two glasses a day) increases longevity.

4. **Nuts**, such as almonds and walnuts, lower cholesterol. Though nuts are high in fat, it is the good kind. Get unsalted nuts so as to avoid excessive salt intake.

5. **Whole-grains** contain anti-cancer agents and help stabilise blood sugar and insulin, which is thought to promote longevity. Eat more whole-grain dark bread, and cereals such as All-Bran and porridge.

6. **Oily fish**, such as salmon, sardines, mackerel, and trout, are high in *omega-3 oil,* which helps us fight disease. It is essential to get some omega-3 oil regularly for the function of the brain, heart, arteries, and joints. Try to get at least two servings a week.

7. **Blueberries**, one of the richest sources of antioxidants, have been proved to stimulate the brain and reverse failing memory. Half a cup of fresh or frozen blueberries a day (or some blueberry jam) is considered to be beneficial.

8. **Garlic** is full of antioxidants, which can protect us from cancer, heart disease, and general ageing. Let crushed or cut garlic 'rest' for about ten minutes before using it in cooking.

9. **Spinach** is also high in antioxidants and rich in folic acid, which helps fight cancer, heart disease, and mental disorders. It can also protect ageing brains from deteriorating.

10. **Tea**, both black and green, has the same beneficial effects as spinach. One cup a day can lower the risk of heart disease.

'Eating right'

Planning a healthy diet may seem complicated and time-consuming. So much information about nutrition and 'miracle' foods is given every week in magazines and newspapers that it may seem impossible to retain all we are told. One day we hear that broccoli is the wonder food, another day onions are declared to be indispensable, or certain vitamins and minerals are found to have the ability to cure nearly every disease on the planet. To help you remember the most important ingredients in a healthy diet for the older person, I will use the 'food pyramid'. If you think of a pyramid, and place food in order of importance from the bottom up, it will help you to understand a healthy diet more clearly.

There are *eight glasses of water* at the bottom of the pyramid. Then come *bread, cereals, rice, and pasta,* of which you should have six or more servings (a bowl of cereal, three slices of bread and two potatoes could be a typical day's ration).

Vegetables and fruit come next, and you should have five or more servings a day of these (a banana, an apple, a tomato, some carrots, and peas).

Milk, yoghurt and cheese (low-fat) are in the following section, with *meat, poultry, fish, eggs, and nuts,* of which you should have two servings a day.

In the smallest section at the top we find *fats, oils, and sweets,* of which you should have only very small amounts.

In addition, a calcium and vitamin D supplement as well as some vitamin B_{12} should be taken every day.

 ## The daily fare

A day's healthy eating could look something like this:

Breakfast

A small bowl of Bran Flakes with low-fat milk

A sliced banana

Two slices of whole-grain toast with low-fat spread (made with olive oil or Benecol)

A glass of orange juice

Mid-morning snack

An apple

One slice of bread with a scraping of low-fat cream cheese

Lunch

A sandwich of two slices of whole-grain bread with tuna, light mayonnaise, tomato, and lettuce

Two pieces of fruit

A glass of low-fat milk

Mid-afternoon snack

A cup of tea with two oatmeal biscuits

Dinner

Two baked potatoes

A piece of grilled chicken breast

Carrots and broccoli

Lettuce-and-tomato salad with olive oil

One glass of wine

Fruit salad

Take a calcium and vitamin D tablet, and remember to drink eight glasses of water a day, *apart from* juice, milk, coffee, and tea.

Why bother?

Pollution is the biggest threat to our health. It is in the air we breathe, the water we drink, and the food we eat. Poisonous fumes are being pumped into the air, industrial and agricultural waste is flowing into lakes and rivers, toxins get into animal feed and are passed into the human food chain, and fruit and vegetables are sprayed with chemicals. It is very difficult to prevent our bodies from being contaminated in some way. You may wonder why you should bother with a healthy diet. What's the point, since we are attacked by pollution whatever we do?

The strongest argument for a healthy diet is that it makes us feel well. In addition, the foods that contain antioxidants can protect us from the bad effects of many toxins. If you buy organic food, or at least make sure you wash and peel all fruit and vegetables, the good effects of a healthy diet will far outweigh the dangers of pollution.

Conclusion

Eating the right food is one of the best ways to make sure our ageing body stays as healthy as possible. It gives us more energy, improves the immune system, and gives us a feeling of well-being. It will even slow down the ageing process.

It is quite easy to get used to a healthy diet once you learn the most important points.

1. Eat a variety of foods, using the food pyramid as a guide.
2. Eat at least five helpings of fruit and vegetables a day.
3. Eat less fat, and try to keep saturated fats to a minimum.
4. Drink eight glasses of water a day.
5. Try to cut down on salt.
6. Drink only a moderate amount of alcohol.
7. Take a calcium and vitamin D tablet every day.
8. Enjoy your food, and try to find healthier versions of your favourite dishes.

If you take the healthy option and gradually change your eating habits for the better, you will very quickly notice a huge improvement in the way you feel. It is also stimulating to try different foods and tastes. Variety is the spice of life!

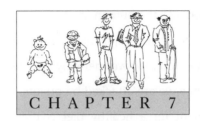

CHAPTER 7

THE BATTLE OF THE BONES
HOW TO PREVENT AND TREAT OSTEOPOROSIS

Osteoporosis, or brittle-bone disease, is often called the silent disease. There are no warning signs in the form of pain or stiffness, and in most cases it is diagnosed when the disease has been present for many years. Osteoporosis mainly affects women but has also been found in men over the age of seventy.

Bone is a dry, dense tissue, 45 per cent mineral (mainly calcium phosphate), 30 per cent organic material, and 25 per cent water. It is constantly breaking down and renewing itself as it supplies many of our organs with calcium. Healthy bone mass appears as a dense network of collagen fibres filled with calcium salts. In a person suffering from osteoporosis the bone mass looks more like a thin mesh; the bones are thin and brittle and fracture easily.

The human skeleton, which is made up of 206 bones, provides the framework for the body. It has several functions: movement, protection (the skull protects the brain, the rib cage protects the heart and lungs), and the supply of calcium to the rest of the body. Individual bones also serve other purposes, such as the attachment of tendons and muscles and the formation of red and white blood cells in the bone marrow.

We reach peak bone mass (when bone is most dense) at the age of thirty and start losing bone around the age of thirty-five. About 80 per cent of bone density is genetically determined, with 20 per cent due to our life-style: how much calcium we take in our diet, how much and what kind of exercise we do, and other factors, such as smoking and alcohol consumption. Twenty per cent may not seem a lot, but doctors maintain that improving bone density by only a few per cent can make the difference between breaking a bone and not.

It is vitally important to detect osteoporosis at the early stage, while bone mass can still be improved.

The risk factors

Certain risk factors are linked to osteoporosis. Most people with the disease have several risk factors, but there are some patients who may have demonstrated none. Some of the risk factors are unmodifiable, others modifiable.

The unmodifiable risk factors are:

Sex: The majority of osteoporosis sufferers are women. Most develop the disease around the menopause, as the depletion of oestrogen affects bone mass.

Age: The older you are, the weaker and less dense your bones. An elderly woman is at a high risk of brittle bones.

Body size: Small, fine-boned women are at greater risk.

Race: White and Asian women have a higher risk of brittle bones than Hispanic and African-American women.

Family history: If you have slight body build and a family member with osteoporosis, the chances are you will develop the disease. Peak bone mass is genetically determined. It is important to find out the medical history of older (especially female) family members to determine your likelihood of being a sufferer.

Premature menopause: The female hormone *oestrogen,* which is present during the reproductive years, protects young women from loss of bone mass. When the menopause occurs before the age of forty-five, naturally or because of the removal of the ovaries or chemotherapy for cancer, it is considered premature. Women who have an early menopause are at greater risk of osteoporosis because of the resulting fall in oestrogen.

Steroid therapy: When cortisone or other steroids are prescribed for conditions such as rheumatic disease, lung disease, inflammation of the bowel or some cancers, it can lead to rapid bone loss and osteoporosis. Short courses and low doses of steroids are not considered harmful, however.

Thyroid disease: Overproduction of *thyroxine,* a hormone produced by the thyroid gland, causes bone loss and subsequent osteoporosis if not treated in time.

Cancer: Some cancers can cause rapid bone loss.

The modifiable risk factors have to do with our life-style. If you are at risk, life-style changes at an early stage may help lessen, or even prevent, the disease. That is why it is important for everyone over forty to be tested for the disease. Knowing the main risk factors can also help early detection. Women in their fifties who have followed this advice have been found to have similar bone density to that of 35-year-olds.

The modifiable (life-style) risk factors are:

Poor diet: A diet low in calcium from childhood can cause a lower peak bone mass (the maximum bone mass at around thirty). Vitamin D deficiency causes softening of the bones and also increases bone loss and the risk of fractures. Women who have been on weight-loss diets usually have a poor intake of calcium, as milk is wrongly thought to be fattening. People suffering from eating disorders, such as bulimia and anorexia, are at high risk. A high intake of protein, caffeine and salt may also increase the risk of osteoporosis.

If you know you are at risk, try to increase the amount of calcium in your daily diet. At about forty and beyond, a daily allowance of 1,200–1,500 mg is recommended. (See chapter 6.)

Alcohol: Moderate amounts of alcohol (see chapter 1) are thought to be beneficial to bone mass. If you exceed the recommended amount, however, it will have the opposite effect. Too much alcohol increases the risk of fractures, both because of reduced bone mass and the risk of falling when intoxicated.

Smoking: Women who smoke tend to have an earlier menopause and lower oestrogen levels than non-smokers. Tobacco is also thought to have a harmful effect on *osteoblasts* (the cells that build bone).

Lack of exercise: It is important to keep physically active all through life. A person who has had a sedentary childhood and adolescence may have reduced peak bone mass. People who have been forced by illness or injury to stay immobile lose bone mass very quickly. Older people who are physically inactive also have poor muscle strength, which can lead to falling and fractures. Taking up weight-bearing exercise, such as walking, will stabilise bone mass and even make bones stronger.

Signs and symptoms

Osteoporosis normally makes itself known when a fracture occurs. Before that, the sufferer would be unaware of the disease (unless he or she had a bone scan). Wrist, spine and hip fractures are the most common, though fractures in other parts of the body also happen, mainly in the pelvis and upper arm.

Spine fractures may result from falling, but they also occur as a result of a sudden movement, coughing, lifting, or turning. There is usually sudden severe pain in the affected vertebra, which can spread to the front of the body. In this kind of fracture the bones do not break; instead there is a change in the shape of the vertebra. The bone becomes thin in one part, which causes it to become compressed. Back pain in elderly women is often caused by compressed vertebrae as a result of osteoporosis. The vertebra never regains its lost bone. A spine fracture can happen to relatively young people who suffer from osteoporosis.

Apart from pain, spine fractures cause a number of other symptoms, such as loss of height and spinal deformity. A bent back, formerly referred to as 'dowager's hump', is the result of fractured or compressed vertebrae caused by loss of bone mass. This causes the chest and abdomen to be pushed downwards, pushing the stomach out. Sometimes the chest is pushed so far down that the lower ribs come into contact with the top of the pelvis, which can be very uncomfortable. This may result in shortness of breath, as there is less room for the lungs to inflate. If the spine is severely deformed, it can be difficult to hold the head up, which may cause neck pain and headaches.

Hip fractures, which mainly affect people around the age of eighty, are a break in the top part of the *femur* (thigh bone), usually as a result of falling from standing height. Old people tend to lean slightly backwards when they walk and so find it difficult to break their fall with their arms. Hip fractures are very painful and require surgery. Sometimes a hip replacement operation—the insertion of an artificial hip joint—is performed. As patients with hip fractures are nearly always elderly and frail, complications are common, and the stay in hospital is often long.

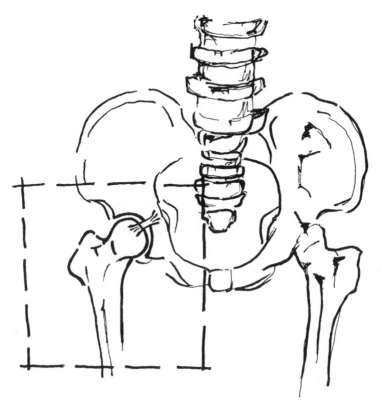

Falling causes fractures

Each year, thousands of older people are injured, and sometimes disabled, by falls that result in broken bones. People who suffer from osteoporosis (and who may, as I pointed out above, be unaware of their condition) are most at risk. About a third of people over sixty-five fall at least once, and half these falls lead to broken bones. This number increases to 50 per cent by the age of eighty. A simple fall can cause a serious change in someone's life.

The reasons older people fall are many, and mostly preventable. Old people are often unfit, with poor muscle strength, balance, and co-ordination. Older people are often on the kinds of medication that impair balance.

Few homes are adapted to reduce the risk of falling. The greatest dangers are caused by the floors, which can be a minefield of hazards: loose rugs, runners and mats, curled carpet edges, electrical flexes, and uncarpeted slippery surfaces. Stairs with no handrails, uneven steps or poor lighting, bathrooms with slippery floors and baths and showers without handrails are also particular sources of danger.

It is quite easy to improve the safety of your home.

~ Install handrails on stairs and grab-rails in baths and showers.

~ Put non-slip rubber mats in baths and showers.

~ Cover the stairs with tightly woven carpet.

~ Use a step-stool with handrails.

~ Do not wax or polish floors, and clean up spills as soon as they happen.

~ Wear low-heeled shoes with non-slip soles. Keep your laces tied.

~ Don't use a bed that is too high. When you are getting up, sit on the edge of the bed for a few minutes, and rise slowly to make sure you are not dizzy.

~ Get rid of loose rugs, or stick them down. Make sure carpets don't curl at the edges.

Prevention is better than cure

It is very important to find out if you are at risk of osteoporosis. As it is a preventable condition, early detection is essential: it can make the difference between strong bones and a comfortable old age and brittle bones and constant fractures, admission to hospital, and chronic pain.

The only way to discover the state of your skeleton is to have a bone scan. Your GP will organise a scan for you at the nearest hospital that has bone-scanning equipment. The newest scanning machines can measure bones in a matter of minutes, instead of the half hour required by older equipment.

Having your bones scanned is a painless and quite comfortable procedure. You lie on a couch; a thin metal arm moves up and down over the site of measurement, and the spine, hip and wrist are measured by x-rays. It is a simple procedure, not requiring you to receive an injection, pass through a tunnel, or even undress. The amount of radiation is minimal, similar to that of a scanner at an airport.

All menopausal women should have this test.

 ## Treatment

No treatment is available that will reverse the effects of osteoporosis once it is established; but a lot can be done to prevent further bone loss and to relieve painful symptoms. The main methods are weight-bearing exercise, an adequate amount of calcium in the diet, and for post-menopausal women, hormone replacement therapy.

Weight-bearing exercise means any exercise that requires the body to support its own weight: walking, running, jumping and skipping are good examples. These exercises will benefit the bones that are taking the strain. It is not only the weight-bearing aspect of the exercise that is important but also the speed and rhythm. This type of exercise stimulates both the cells that build bones and the production of growth hormones, which help improve bone mass.

Walking briskly for thirty minutes three or four times a week will reduce bone loss in hips and spine in older women. Badminton, tennis and golf are excellent sports, as they require in addition a certain degree of skill, such as co-ordination and balance, that can help prevent falls in the home.

Recent studies show that muscle-strengthening exercises with weights also have a beneficial effect on bones, as do other sports, such as cycling and horse-riding. When we exercise, the muscles pull on the bones, thus stimulating them to make more bone tissue.

Get advice from an instructor if you are going to use weights. Avoid exercises that involve bending forward or twisting the spine, as this can cause further fractures of the vertebrae. Ask your doctor for advice on which exercise is suitable for you, as weak bones may not be able to take the strain of vigorous exercise too soon.

Diets have to contain enough calcium and vitamin D to maintain strong bones. (Chapter 6 described such a diet and showed you the amount of calcium that should be taken every day.) If you take calcium supplements, do take them in several small doses, as the body cannot absorb large quantities at once. It's better to drink a glass of milk at breakfast, lunch and dinner than three glasses at once.

It has to be said, however, that taking large amounts of calcium will have little or no effect if it is not combined with exercise (and vice versa).

Hormone replacement therapy (HRT) has been used for many years to treat osteoporosis in post-menopausal women. It prevents bone loss during and after the menopause and reduces the risk of fractures; it is also effective in women in their sixties and seventies. It involves treatment with either oestrogen alone or a combination of oestrogen and progesterone. Both hormones are produced by the ovaries, and the level declines during the menopause.

HRT may be taken by mouth, as a skin patch, or as an implant under the skin. It may be necessary to take HRT for the rest of your life to keep the protection against osteoporosis.

Some women are unable to take hormones, either because of side-effects or a family history of breast cancer. In that case there are several alternatives, in the form of synthetic drugs that deactivate the bone-destroying cells (*osteoclasts*), thus preventing bone loss. There are two types: Etidronate and Alendronate. They have to be taken with calcium supplements and have few side-effects. Other drugs are also available, which your doctor can advise you about.

Recent research shows that a diet rich in soya can promote the growth of new bone cells, which may help prevent osteoporosis. Soya has long been thought to act as a natural hormone, with the same effects as the body's own hormones. Some countries where diets are high in soya products, such as Japan and China, have a much lower rate of hip fractures than western countries. Including soya products in your diet can also help alleviate many menopausal symptoms. A glass of soya milk (with added calcium) per day will give you a good supply of soya.

Managing pain

The pain associated with osteoporosis varies from patient to patient. Some have severe and chronic pain, others only minor discomfort. Pain after hip or wrist fractures usually improves after surgery.

Patients with spinal fractures sometimes have pain that is difficult to treat. Bed rest may be necessary for a time, but this should be kept to a minimum, as rest can cause further bone loss. There are several types of drugs that may help, which will be administered on the advice of the doctor in charge.

Treating pain with heat can help some people: try heat pads or a hot-water bottle. In other cases, ice packs have proved useful, as has acupuncture. A method called *transcutaneous electrical nerve stimulation* (TENS), which involves attaching electrodes to the painful area, causing a tingling sensation, has been shown to be helpful for some patients.

Physiotherapy is very useful in treating the symptoms of osteoporosis with exercise, relieving pain and discomfort and improving mobility. With spinal fractures, the muscles around the affected vertebra often tense and go into spasm, causing more pain. Gentle manipulation will relieve pain by relaxing the muscles. *Hydrotherapy* (exercise in warm water) is another way of relaxing muscles, which is pleasant and soothing. Both physiotherapy and hydrotherapy can help restore confidence in patients who have had fractures and may be afraid to move about in case it will cause further damage.

Comfortable chairs with support cushions for the lower back, and firm beds, are also ways of reducing discomfort and making daily life more bearable.

Osteoporosis in men

Osteoporosis is generally regarded as a women's affliction; but recent studies reveal that men are also affected. It is difficult to ascertain how to treat the disease in men, as there appears to be little knowledge about it at present.

A deficiency in the male hormone *testosterone* is sometimes found in men with osteoporosis. Testosterone acts on bones in a similar way to oestrogen in women. It should be given in synthetic form to men with brittle bones. Vitamin D supplements and calcium should also be taken in a similar way to women.

Men over sixty-five should have their bone density tested. Recent research shows that osteoporosis in elderly men is far more common than was previously thought.

Conclusion

Our bone mass has a short life and needs a constant supply of calcium. Paying attention to calcium in our diet, making our bones strong with the right type of exercise and finding out about the state of our skeleton with a bone scan are the best ways to prevent, or in any case to slow down, osteoporosis.

If you remember a few simple rules, you can make sure of strong bones for the rest of your life.

~ Make sure you get at least 1,200 mg of calcium daily. (One glass of milk provides about 250 mg, skim milk a little more.)

~ Go outdoors. Vitamin D (produced in the skin by sunlight) is essential for the absorption of calcium and also prevents it being lost by way of our kidneys.

~ Take weight-bearing exercise three or four times a week for about thirty minutes.

~ Stop smoking, and cut down on alcohol.

~ Eat soya products, such as tofu, soya milk, beans, and pulses, which protect us against bone loss.

~ Arrange with your doctor to have a bone scan. Early detection is important to prevent further bone loss.

There is no other treatment for osteoporosis. But consider the fringe benefits in the form of general well-being!

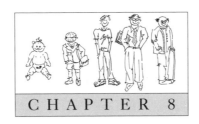

CHAPTER 8

CREAKING JOINTS AND ACHING BONES
KEEPING STRONG AND SUPPLE

Sore, stiff joints, aching muscles and a less-than-supple body are some of the most annoying signs of ageing. Even the very fit feel the effects of growing older: they too can wake up in the morning feeling in need of a can of oil.

Stiffness is often taken as a signal to stop physical activities. It seems more comfortable to adopt a sedentary life-style than to keep active. It's very tempting to soothe aching joints and stiff muscles by sitting in a comfortable chair, or lying in a soft bed, while reading or watching television. Cushions, shawls and slippers replace running-shoes, tennis rackets, and golf clubs.

Your doctor diagnoses either arthritis or rheumatism, or both. Is this the beginning of an uncomfortable old age? Not if you don't want it to be!

While it's true that few older people escape some degree of aches and pains, there are ways of keeping mobile and relatively free of pain throughout life. Picking the right parents can certainly help, as genes play an important role in the way our joints cope with ageing (30 per cent of osteo-arthritis in the hand and 65 per cent in the knees is of genetic origin); but a healthy diet and life-style are also important.

In this chapter I explain aching joints and stiff muscles, what causes them, and what can be done to alleviate the worst discomforts.

~
99

Joints

Our body's framework, the skeletal system, is made up of bones that are connected at our joints. These consist of three types: fixed joints, slightly movable joints, and freely movable joints.

Fixed joints provide no movement, as for example the joins between the bones of the skull.

Slightly movable joints are found in the pelvis, *sacro-iliac joint* (lower back), and both ends of the *clavicle* (collar bone). These bones are held together by strong *ligaments* and are separated by pads of *cartilage,* which act as shock-absorbers.

Freely movable joints (*synovial joints*) are enclosed in a fibrous capsule, supported by ligaments. This capsule is lined with a *synovial membrane* with *synovial fluid* in the cavity. This fluid, whitish and similar to egg-white in consistency, acts like oil in a machine to reduce friction between the moving surfaces in the joint. The bone surfaces are covered with *hyaline cartilage,* which is smooth to ensure friction-free movement.

There are four main groups of freely movable joints:

~ ball-and-socket joint (hip and shoulder)

~ hinge joint (knee and elbow)

~ pivot joint (the *radius* and *ulna* in the lower arm, and the *cervical joints* in the neck)

~ gliding joint (ankle and wrist).

Joints are connected and moved by *soft tissue*: muscles, tendons, and ligaments. Some muscles are attached directly to the bone; others are attached to the bone by tendons. Ligaments attach bone to bone.

Synovial membranes are present in parts of the body other than synovial joints. When this tissue is between the bone and a muscle, or between two muscles, it is called a *bursa.* It forms a little enclosed sac of fluid that allows tissues to run over each other in a smooth way. Bursae allow the body to move smoothly by lubricating rough surfaces; they are mostly around the shoulder, hip and knee joints, but also in other parts of the body. This membrane can become inflamed with overuse, which may result in a condition known as *bursitis* (so-called 'housemaid's knee' is one example).

Our joints can be affected by several conditions, most of which are referred to as *rheumatism*, which can affect either the skeletal system or the muscular system. *Arthritis* affects the joints, and *fibrositis* is a disease of the muscular system.

Arthritis

Arthritis is inflammation of a joint. There are two types: *inflammatory arthritis* (which includes rheumatoid arthritis and gout) and *osteo-arthritis*. Both result in swollen, stiff joints; but that is the only thing they have in common.

Rheumatoid arthritis is the most common form of inflammatory arthritis. It is a long-term disease that affects the synovial membrane lining the joints. It has nothing to do with ageing: you can get it at any age, and it most commonly strikes in the mid-thirties or early forties. Rheumatoid arthritis causes inflammation of the joints, tendon sheaths, muscles, and bursae. The synovial membrane becomes inflamed, with white blood cells accumulating in the affected area, causing the joint to swell. The cartilage becomes covered by inflamed synovial tissue, which eventually destroys it.

The cause of this disease is not known, but it is thought to be connected with changes in the immune system when the body is attacked by a virus or other infection. There is also a genetic link: those with a brother or sister who has the disease have five times the risk of the general population.

The symptoms of rheumatoid arthritis include swelling, stiffness, and pain, which often starts in a symmetrical fashion, affecting both sides of the body at once. It is usually the hands and wrists that are affected at first, with the condition gradually spreading to other joints, such as the elbows, shoulders, and ankles. The symptoms vary in severity from day to day; the persistent inflammation often lasts six weeks or more.

Rheumatoid arthritis can be diagnosed by a blood test, which will confirm the presence of the rheumatoid factor antibody. Some patients with rheumatoid arthritis do not have this antibody in their blood; in that case the disease has to be diagnosed by a combination of blood tests that will disclose inflammation.

The treatments for rheumatoid arthritis are many and varied. There is no cure, and therapies include drugs, injections, physiotherapy, hydrotherapy, and special exercises. No single method is universally successful, as the illness varies in severity from patient to patient. It can also worsen with age.

Osteo-arthritis is the most common form of joint damage. Unlike rheumatoid arthritis, it is the most prevalent sign of ageing, and all old people are affected by it to a greater or lesser degree.

Most stiffness and pain we feel as we age (other than that resulting from strenuous exercise) is due to osteo-arthritis. It is a condition that affects *cartilage,* the gristle material that covers the ends of bones and forms the smooth surface of the joint on both sides. Cartilage is tough, quite elastic, and very durable. It does not have a blood supply and gets its oxygen and nutrients from the joint fluid. When we use a joint by moving it, the pressure squeezes fluid and waste products out of the cartilage; and when we relax the fluid seeps back, with oxygen and nutrients. *That is why the elasticity of cartilage depends on how much we use a joint.* Physical activity, therefore, helps keep our joints supple.

As we age, the cartilage protecting the ends of the bones gradually flakes off, leaving the bones to grate on each other, causing damage to the surface of the bone. As a result, the bones start getting thicker, and new lumpy bone develops at the sides of the joint. In most cases the resulting osteo-arthritis is not serious enough to cause more than a little discomfort, with stiffness and mild pain from time to time.

❭ Wear and tear

The usual description of arthritis as 'wear and tear' is not accurate. Careful studies of people who have put a lot of strain on their joints have been unable to show joint damage as a result of these activities—on the contrary, activity helps keep joints supple and lubricated.

The joints most affected by osteo-arthritis are those exposed to weight-bearing: the spine, knees, and hips. In women, the fingers and thumbs are also in danger, as these joints are finer than men's. The gnarled appearance of older people's fingers is due to osteo-arthritis. Arthritis can also be caused by trauma: the joint may have been damaged at some time in an accident or a sports injury.

Even though we will all have some form of wear and tear in our joints as we age, severe arthritis with resulting pain and discomfort is not inevitable. Fortunately, osteo-arthritis is usually a mild condition and only rarely causes severe symptoms. Mild forms of arthritis do not cause any symptoms and are only discovered by an x-ray. In more severe arthritis, damage to the joint is serious enough to cause considerable pain and stiffness. It can develop mainly after middle age, and women are more prone to it than men, because of their weaker joint structure. Being overweight also greatly increases the risk: the heavier you are, the greater the load your body has to carry.

The most common symptom is localised pain, which happens mainly with movement. At rest there is usually no pain, but inactivity will cause stiffness, which is most noticeable first thing in the morning. Only in the most advanced cases does the disease cause enough pain to keep you awake.

The pain and stiffness of osteo-arthritis increase gradually over a long time. It can be many years before the odd twinge becomes so painful that you see a doctor. An x-ray will then confirm the condition and show the extent of the damage. Early diagnosis may prevent the disease from becoming too severe, as an exercise routine and certain life-style changes can be very helpful.

Most arthritis sufferers find that the degree of discomfort varies from time to time. Even in severe cases there are periods when the symptoms are hardly felt, and then there are spells of very bad pain.

) The forms of osteo-arthritis

There are three types of osteo-arthritis. The mildest form is that causing changes in the fingers (as described above) with the knobbly enlargement of the finger joints. This form of arthritis usually only causes some stiffness and does not involve any pain.

The second form of arthritis affects the spine, where bony growth appears on the vertebrae of the neck region or further down the back. The discs between the vertebrae are affected. Arthritis of the spine does not cause any symptoms unless there is pressure on a nerve or irritation of some other part of the back, which can cause some pain, discomfort, and stiffness.

The third form of the condition involves the weight-bearing joints and almost always the hips and knees. This form of arthritis develops slowly and often involves both sides of the body. Pain may remain quite constant, or vary in intensity over a number of years. Fluid may accumulate in the affected joint, making it swell or wobble (mainly knee joints) when subjected to weight. In the knee, the arthritis may affect only part of the joint, either the inner or the outer part. This can have the effect of making the leg become bowed or splayed. Walking may become difficult.

It is possible to have two or all three types of osteo-arthritis, though most people suffer only from one.

) Treatment

When osteo-arthritis is diagnosed, your doctor may refer you to a rheumatologist, a specialist in joint disorders, who will prescribe the best treatment for you. Osteo-arthritis is usually treated with some combination of drugs, injections, surgery, and exercise.

Drug therapy is not usually thought to be helpful with osteo-arthritis. It is used to control pain, but as there is little inflammation in this kind of arthritis, drugs with anti-inflammatory properties do not help much. If the osteo-arthritis is in the hip or knee, however, anti-inflammatory drugs may be helpful. Doctors try to avoid strong pain-killers containing codein, because pain is a signal that helps us protect a diseased joint, and it is important that the signal is received.

Injections with corticosteroids into the joint are sometimes helpful. The removal of fluid can also work. Again, injections are not much use to a joint where no inflammation is present. In any case, injections must not be repeated too often, as they may damage cartilage.

Severe osteo-arthritis in the hips or knees is often treated with surgery, which can be dramatically effective for patients with badly damaged joints. Hip surgery is the most important form of surgery for arthritis and can make a huge difference in a sufferer's life. Practically all patients are free of pain afterwards, and most walk normally and can take up normal activities. Total knee replacement has been shown to give better results than the knee surgery available a few years ago, and is nearly as successful as a hip replacement.

You will decide with your doctor at what point surgery is needed to relieve pain and discomfort and to give you back mobility. As this type of surgery is not urgent, you have plenty of time to discuss when surgery is needed, and what type.

Exercise has been found to be the best way to treat deteriorating joints. Many people see the onset of osteo-arthritis as a signal to stop physical activities and slow down their life-style; some think exercise is actually harmful. This is not so. Inactivity will speed up the development of further pain and discomfort. Others may become discouraged because exercise can hurt at first, and progress is slow. It is important to keep muscles and ligaments strong to support joints. Movement is also essential for keeping cartilage supple. If cartilage has been so badly worn away that there is practically none left, moving a joint regularly can polish the bone (a process called *eburnation*) and thus improve mobility.

Numerous studies, including medical research done in hospitals, confirm the importance of exercise. In a recent survey in Britain it was discovered that 95 per cent of arthritis sufferers were helped by daily exercise.

Arthritis exercise has three important ingredients:

~ **Aerobic activities**, such as walking, cycling, and swimming, build stamina and improve cardiovascular (heart and circulation) fitness. They are also easy, can be gradually increased in intensity and speed, and are smooth in action rather than jerky.

~ **Stretching**, or 'range of motion' exercises, such as leg raises and finger curls, keep joints supple and mobile.

~ **Strengthening exercises**, including lifting light weights, will prevent *atrophy* (shrinking) of the muscles.

Each type of exercise plays an important role in maintaining and improving flexibility and also helps prevent the deformities caused by arthritis. Your doctor may refer you to a physiotherapist, who will design a daily exercise routine that suits you and your specific problem.

A number of books are also available with good exercise routines for arthritis. *Arthritis: What Exercises Really Work* by Dava Sobel and Arthur Klein (Robinson) and *The Arthritis Helpbook* by Kate Lorig and James Fries (Souvenir Press) have helped many people. They are full of advice and show detailed exercise programmes, with easy-to-follow instructions.

A good exercise programme will give you a general sense of well-being as you get fitter, apart from the benefits for your joints. It will also increase your confidence as you succeed in maintaining a good exercise routine. It will prevent the loss of function that often comes with arthritis. If you are realistic and don't expect miracles at once, your exercise programme will improve your quality of life, and you will feel well and happy.

Though exercising can be a little uncomfortable, even painful at times, it is essential to move all the joints every day. Remember: if you don't use a muscle or joint, you will lose mobility and strength, and so lose function.

How to exercise

~ Exercise every day, and choose the time of day that suits you best. Osteo-arthritis patients usually prefer to exercise in the morning, as this is the time of day when they have least pain.

~ Don't exercise painful or swollen joints; rest them until the inflammation has gone down.

~ Don't put too much pressure on painful joints; exercise gently, making sure the joint is moved through its full range of motion.

~ Start gently, warming up slowly. That way you can find out how much you can do without too much pain.

~ Little and often is better than doing a lot only occasionally.

~ Don't take medication to mask pain. Instead, slow down a little until the worst pain recedes.

~ Don't stop exercise during 'flare-ups' (periods when pain gets worse), but modify your routine during this time. (Exercise does not cause flare-ups.)

~ Avoid becoming chilled during exercise. Warmth helps relax stiff muscles and joints. Wear warm clothes, and exercise in a heated room. Hand exercises can be done in a basin of warm water.

Diet, supplements, and 'miracle cures'

A healthy diet, low in fat and rich in fruit and vegetables, is essential for good health and a reasonably slim body. Keeping your weight down is one way to prevent your joints from deteriorating too quickly. But no special foods or diets can prevent or cure arthritis. Diet 'cures' are found regularly in magazines and books, which try to make people believe that arthritis can be made to disappear by certain foods.

Surveys show that people who try these diets do not feel any better than those who do not.

Contrary to widespread belief, fish oil does not 'lubricate' joints; but it does have anti-inflammatory properties. Evening primrose oil also reduces inflammation and can help reduce the need for drugs, but it has to be taken over a long period to have any effect. Other supplements that are supposed to be beneficial include collagen and selenium. The problem with these supplements is that so far there is no proof that they have any effect on damaged joints; and they are very expensive.

New research shows that the female hormone *oestrogen* promotes healthy joints in women. Hormone replacement therapy (HRT) can significantly reduce the risk of osteo-arthritis in post-menopausal women, particularly in the knees.

Glucosamine is a natural substance found in the human body. As we age, we lose a large amount of glucosamine in the connective tissue (muscles, tendons, ligaments, bone, and cartilage), which causes cartilage to become thinner. In clinical trials, glucosamine taken orally reversed degenerative osteo-arthritis of the knee after two months. In animal studies it raised blood sugar; so diabetes sufferers should not take it without consulting their doctor. The research is still in its infancy, and there is little information on the long-term benefits, or indeed risks, of glucosamine.

Any so-called 'natural' ingredient powerful enough to have an effect on the symptoms of osteo-arthritis may be risky to take in large amounts. Many herbs and other remedies available in health food shops are not subjected to checks in the way that medicines are. *Do not take any remedy without asking your doctor for advice.*

❭ Heat treatment

The discomfort of osteo-arthritis can be alleviated by heat. Pain in the hands can be relieved with hot soaks and warm paraffin. Pains in the hips can be treated with heating pads or *diathermy,* which uses a mild electric current to produce heat. Infra-red light therapy has been found to relieve pain in the knees of some sufferers.

Moving to a warmer climate has *not* been found to help arthritis sufferers a great deal. In fact people who live in warmer countries have been found to be more sensitive to changes in temperature than inhabitants of countries with a cold, damp climate.

Mechanical aids

A wide variety of devices can help you support and protect joints. Shock-absorbing soles in your shoes can help to make walking more comfortable. Splints or braces help align joints and distribute weight properly; these are made of lightweight metal, leather, foam, and plastic, with Velcro straps.

There are also a number of gadgets designed to make housework easier. Special versions of household tools such as peelers, can-openers, scissors and many others help prevent too much strain on sore joints. Don't hesitate to use a device that can make daily life a little easier. It is important to avoid too much stress on arthritic joints by lifting heavy loads, bending, or twisting.

If you suffer from arthritis, protect your joints by

~ avoiding heavy lifting or gripping; always use two hands whenever possible

~ adjusting the height of your bed and chair so they are easy to get out of

~ trying not to go up and down stairs unnecessarily

~ choosing shoes that are easy to put on and take off

~ pacing yourself: instead of doing all the ironing, gardening or tidying at once, do a little each day.

Prevention

Doctors now believe osteo-arthritis may be prevented by the right life-style. If you are physically active, keep your weight down, exercise your muscles and joints regularly in order to keep cartilage nourished and elastic, and don't keep up exercise that is too strenuous or painful, your joints should last a lifetime.

❭ Prognosis

The prognosis for osteo-arthritis is very good. The condition develops slowly over many years, and there is much that can be done to slow down the deterioration of your joints. It is very rarely a crippling condition, and with a little care and attention you can remain free of symptoms for most of your life.

Muscular pain

Pain and stiffness in and around the joints can have causes other than arthritis. *Fibrositis* or *fibromyalgia* is a disease of the muscular system where there is a build-up of urea and *lactic acid* (waste products) inside the muscle, causing pain similar to that of arthritis. There can also be inflammation. The excessive amount of waste product in the muscles is caused by too much exercise, stress, or tension, or by an injury or a viral infection. The waste products are deposited between the muscle fibres, which makes them swell and press on nerves. If fibrositis is caused by an injury, the pain continues even after the injury heals.

Fibrositis is the most common cause of chronic rheumatic complaints. It is present in all ages but is most common in women in the 20–50 age group. It is not usual for older people to get fibrositis suddenly, but milder problems that are present for many·years worsen in later life. Fibrositis is often referred to as rheumatism, or *non-articular rheumatism.*

Well-known examples of fibrositis include *lumbago,* which causes lower-back pain, and *torticollis* or 'wry neck', when there is stiffness, pain and reduced function in one side of the neck. There can also be chronic pain, especially in the lower back and neck area, usually caused by adopting the wrong position for long periods. A visit to a specialist, who, with a little detective work, can find out the cause, will do a great deal to solve the problem. It could be your bed, your pillow or your chair that forces you into the wrong position. You could be standing, sitting or walking in way that puts uneven stress on the muscles and tendons, causing inflammation or just strain.

The main symptoms of fibrositis are pain and stiffness. The pain can be severe but is more likely to be a dull aching or a sensation of burning. The stiffness is usually worse in the morning and is often eased by movement or heat. Other signs of fibrositis are fluid retention and puffiness or swelling of the hands. Your rings may tighten, and your grip may be weaker. There may even be pins and needles, tingling or numbness in your hands.

Fatigue is also quite a common problem for people with fibrositis. This can vary through the day, the week, or over many months.

The symptoms can be absent for a long time, only to reappear suddenly as a result of a change in the weather, physical activity, or emotional stress. Humid weather seems to make the condition worse; dry weather, even if it is cold, has a beneficial effect.

Unaccustomed vigorous activity, such as a burst of house-cleaning or gardening, can also stir up symptoms, as can sitting or standing in an awkward position for a long time. (I suffered from chronic lower-back pain until I changed the hard kitchen chair I used while working on the computer for a proper office chair. The improvement was dramatic.) Emotional stress can cause you to tense your muscles in a particular area.

Fibrositis is treated with anti-inflammatory drugs and exercise. Pain-killers decrease severe pain and inflammation. Exercise reduces stress, improves circulation, eases stiffness, and increases strength and flexibility in joints and muscles.

With an acute flare-up of pain you might try either ice or heat. Some people find great relief in applying an ice-pack to the painful area: a packet of frozen peas from the freezer, wrapped in a towel, can be put on the sore area for twenty minutes.

Some find heat very soothing. If ice is not comfortable, try a hot-water bottle wrapped in a towel for the same amount of time.

Other forms of treatment include physical therapy, acupuncture, massage, and transcutaneous electrical nerve stimulation (TENS), which should be used in addition to fitness training and relaxation.

As with any kind of muscle or joint pain, it is best to get medical advice before embarking on an exercise routine. When you have the correct diagnosis of your particular type of rheumatism you will know what kind of exercises you should, and should not, do. In any fitness programme it is important to start slowly, building up strength and stamina gradually.

Lower-back pain

Very few people avoid some sort of lower-back pain at some time in their life. The lower back is subjected to enormous stress all through life, and all older people have some sort of wear-and-tear damage in that region. Lower-back pain is a significant health care problem; it is also the most difficult complaint to diagnose and cure.

The spine consists of thirty-three *vertebrae,* twenty-four of which are movable and separated by pads of *fibrocartilage.* The last nine vertebrae are fixed—they are fused together, with no movement between them, except for the *coccyx,* which moves with the *sacrum* (the lowest joint of the back).

The discs between the vertebrae act both like cushions and like ball bearings, allowing the spine to twist and bend. A network of ligaments holds the spine together, and a range of muscles controls posture and movement.

There are a number of disorders that cause back pain, such as *prolapsed* or 'slipped' disc, rheumatic arthritis and osteo-arthritis, osteoporosis, spondylosis (a degenerative disease of the spine), and fibrositis.

Acute back pain is often no more than a strained muscle. Most cases of acute back pain usually clear up after a few days or a week without any further damage; but some people develop chronic problems, with pain that comes and goes from day to day or from week to week.

Back pain in older people is mostly caused, however, by osteo-arthritis or osteoporosis. In an arthritis sufferer, the pain is caused by the degeneration of the discs between the vertebrae. In osteoporosis, compressed vertebrae are the source of most pain (as explained in chapter 7). In both cases, pain can be greatly alleviated by exercise. Taking care of your back by not twisting, bending or lifting heavy loads will prevent further damage.

Chronic back pain can also be caused by bad posture, and by beds or chairs that are either too soft or too hard. People who are overweight are more prone to backache, because of the strain on their spine. In any case, it is important to seek medical advice for any back pain that lasts longer than a week. Your doctor will refer you to a physiotherapist, who will advise you and teach you how to exercise, correct bad posture, and choose furniture more suitable for older backs.

Severe back pain is not inevitable as you age: most cases of lower-back problems can be improved with proper care.

Aching knees

Ageing athletes wearing knee braces are a common sight these days. You see them on ski slopes, on tennis courts, and in marathons. It is normal to assume that exercise ruins your knees. In our ageing society, damaged knees are a big concern; they are becoming nearly as common as back pain.

The knee is the largest joint in the body and the only one that forms a full hinge: the bones are able to move both forward and backwards. The *patella,* or kneecap, fits into the hinge like a wedge, preventing the lower leg from coming too far forward. It is a complex joint, used for a wide variety of functions, including walking, running, jumping, kneeling, and kicking. And it is the most easily injured. Structural imbalance, which can be present from birth, such as uneven legs or 'knock-knees', can cause uneven wear on the joint. This type of imperfection can be corrected with special shoes, which will reduce the stress on the joint.

Many knee injuries occur during everyday activities. Some happen during exercise: sports such as soccer, basketball, skiing, jogging and rugby are hard on the knees, because they involve movements like twisting, changing direction quickly, slowing down when running, and jumping. Running, long associated with knee injury, is not in itself too hard on the knees but can cause damage over time.

As more and more people continue practising sports at a high intensity at quite an advanced age, the increase in the number of people with arthritic knees is destined to rise dramatically.

The answer is *not* to stop exercising. Maintaining strength, flexibility and a reasonable weight is essential to healthy knees (and a healthy body). Instead, it is important to take care of any sports injury, rehabilitate it, and correct any imbalance with shoe inserts, strengthening exercises, and stretching. This will also reduce the risk of further problems.

Some people try to run through an injury. This is wrong. If you feel a sharp, sustained pain, stop exercising at once and seek treatment. If the pain is dull and nagging, take a few days off and try to work out the cause. Do you need new shoes? Have you been doing something different? If the pain doesn't go away with self-treatment (ice and rest), seek professional help.

It is also important to pick a sport that is right for your body. Some people are not biomechanically designed for running. If you have wide hips or knock-knees, you are at a greater risk of developing knee problems. Try walking instead. If the sport you are involved in makes your knees ache, switch to something else. In any case, it is better to vary your fitness routine by alternating activities. Try swimming one day and walking the following day; you will reduce the risk of overusing a particular joint.

Eight tips for healthy knees

1. Never lock your knees: keep them 'soft', or slightly bent.

2. Keep hip, knee and ankle in alignment. Do not bow your knees in or out.

3. Strengthen muscles that are weak, and stretch muscles that are tight. Tight hamstrings and weak *quadriceps* (the muscle in front of the thigh attached to your kneecap) are often the cause of knee problems.

4. Avoid twisting on a planted foot or doing full squats or lunges in which knees extend out over your toes.

5. Wear the right shoes for your activity.

6. Keep your weight down, to avoid excess strain on your knees.

7. 'Cross-train' by alternating your activities.

8. Do not try to play sports to get fit. Get fit to play sports.

If you are careful and follow this advice, your knees should stay in good shape all through your life.

 # Conclusion

Though no-one escapes a certain amount of stiffness and aching in joints and muscles as they get older, it is important to remember that daily physical activity is far better than sitting still. Sports can make you stiff and sore from time to time, but doing nothing will make you feel even worse.

It is true that our muscles, tendons and ligaments lose their elasticity with age. But it is also true that we can slow down this process by moving every part of our body regularly. It is the only way to stay reasonably pain-free. The less you do, the more you will ache.

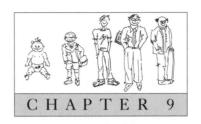

CHAPTER 9

COMING OUT OF THE DARK
HOW TO DEAL WITH DEPRESSION

Depression is one of the most common problems among the elderly. It is not an inevitable part of ageing, as it can affect anyone at any age, but it often goes undiagnosed in older people.

Depression is a term used for many mood disorders, from being 'down in the dumps' to feeling suicidal. But in reality it is more than feeling sad or a bit down. A person suffering from clinical depression has usually lost interest in life, is not sleeping, and has little energy or appetite.

Depression affects a large number of elderly people. Older people often have to cope with tremendous hardships, such as bereavement, loneliness, illness, and financial problems. As we age, it is also difficult to face the fact that we can no loner manage to do as much as we did when we were younger. It is hardly surprising that many older people become depressed.

Older people do not seek psychiatric help as readily as younger people do. This is partly because seeking counselling may label them as mentally ill, partly because they do not know how to seek help.

Why we get depressed

Depression is usually the result of stress affecting the vulnerable part of a person's personality. Early life experiences, poor self-image, social circumstances and biological factors can play a role.

When a person is depressed, chemical changes in the brain take place. *Neurotransmitters* carry nerve impulses from one nerve cell to another. If some of them are underactive or carry too few impulses, the result is depression. There can be problems in the manufacture, storage or release of the neurotransmitter as well. These processes are often triggered by negative life events, but in some people it happens for no obvious reason.

Certain individuals are prone to depression because of a sensitivity they have inherited. Our genes control the chemical processes that occur in the brain, and there are indications that a malfunction in the way neurochemicals are produced can lead to depression.

Women are more likely than men to suffer from depression. It is not really known why, but one possibility is that fluctuating hormone levels make them more susceptible.

Traumas such as bereavement, illness, financial difficulties and sudden loneliness because of the loss of a partner, or because of children leaving home, can trigger depression. Poor living conditions, chronic pain or illness and moving from home to a nursing-home are other examples.

 # How to detect depression

Depression is not simply feeling sad. There are difficult times for everyone all through life, and it is normal to feel sad at those times. The sadness caused by a life event—for example the death of someone we love—is called *reactive depression.* It normally lessens with time. The depression of the elderly is often *endogenous depression,* coming from within. It either starts for no specific reason or lingers long

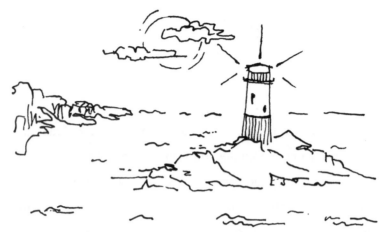

after an unhappy event, when a reactive depression would have passed. Certain illnesses or drugs can also cause the symptoms of depression.

Detecting depression in an older person can be complicated by several factors. Often symptoms, such as fatigue, loss of appetite, and difficulties with sleeping, are thought to be part of the ageing process. But it is not normal to feel depressed all the time when you get older. An older person who is showing signs of depression should seek medical help. Being old does not mean feeling sad and down all the time.

A person may be suffering from clinical depression if he or she

~ is depressed or irritable

~ has lost interest in daily activities

~ gets angry or agitated about minor things

~ loses appetite

~ either loses or gains weight unintentionally

~ sleeps either too little or too much

~ has feelings of worthlessness

~ experiences memory loss

~ has abnormal thoughts, including excessive guilt

~ has thoughts about suicide.

Each person will experience a different combination of symptoms, and these may also vary in severity. For some the symptoms are mainly physical, for others emotional. Whatever the causes, depression makes the sufferer feel confused, frightened, isolated, and lonely.

Depression and its symptoms vary in severity. It can be mild, moderate, or severe. Mild and moderate depression are characterised by negative thinking, low self-esteem, irritability, and difficulties in concentrating. This low-grade form of depression usually lasts for a year or more and can easily go undetected.

Severe or major depression is usually more dramatic, and the same symptoms are more intense and usually accompanied by physical manifestations. Changes in sleeping patterns, loss of appetite, weight gain or loss and a noticeable change in both physical and mental activities call for medical help. In particular, thoughts of suicide must always be taken seriously.

Severe depression is usually diagnosed if the majority of the symptoms described above are present every day for a period of at least two weeks.

 ## Other forms of depression

Other types of depression that can show the same symptoms, but demand different treatments, are seasonal affective disorder and manic depression.

Seasonal affective disorder (SAD) is a condition that involves recurring episodes of depression during autumn and winter, caused by a lack of light. The symptoms include weight gain because of increased appetite and carbohydrate cravings, and excessive sleeping, which usually starts in October or November and is relieved in the spring. The symptoms ease during sunny days or if the patient spends some time in well-lit areas. Most sufferers experience a worsening in their condition if they move further north, where the winter is longer.

Sitting in front of a bank of bright lights for a time each day relieves the depression. This is thought to be linked to increases in certain hormones in the blood and brain. It is looking at the lights that works, not the effect of the light on the skin. For best results, the patient should sit in front of a bank of 40-watt full-spectrum lights (which is the equivalent of looking out of a window on a sunny day), looking at the lights for a few seconds every few minutes. Four hours of daily treatment in two two-hour sessions, which should be continued until spring, are usually recommended.

Manic depression is a condition that causes violent mood swings. Periods of abnormal elation, excessive physical activity and rapid speech are replaced by moments of severe depression. This type of disorder is thought to be mainly caused by an inherited neurochemical imbalance in the brain and is usually successfully treated with specific medication.

Overcoming depression

Depression is sometimes called the 'common cold of psychiatry', because of its prevalence. It is, however, one of the easiest conditions to treat; but the sufferer must first seek help. The problem with depression is that many people do not go to their doctor when they are feeling depressed. They may feel they can deal with the problem themselves, or they are embarrassed about talking to a doctor about their feelings. Older people in particular tend to think that depression will go away of itself and that they are, in any case, too old to get help. They may even think that looking for help is a sign of weakness or moral failing, or, even worse, of mental illness. Some sufferers have such a strong feeling of hopelessness that they do not believe there is any solution to their condition.

The good news is that even the most seriously depressed person can be treated successfully, often in a matter of weeks, and returned to a happier, more fulfilling life.

To cure depression, however, you must first recognise that you have a problem. If you have two or more of the symptoms mentioned above for more than a few weeks, or if you are feeling worthless or hopeless, or you are crying frequently, go to your doctor, who will refer you to a specialist, therapist, or counsellor. If you are suffering from mild depression, your GP may prescribe medication and other types of treatment.

Medication is now available that identifies the areas in the brain where there is a lack of certain neurotransmitters. Some medication increases the supply of *serotonin,* which can directly affect the negative moods that come with depression; other antidepressants are aimed at other areas involving different neurotransmitters, each with its own benefits according to the symptoms in each individual.

Many doctors now believe that treatment should begin with medication to change the physical chemistry of the brain, especially when there is a family history of depression.

Some people are worried that taking medicine will make them dependent. The advantage of medication, however, is that it may relieve symptoms in a very short time. It can act as a lifebelt in some cases, making it easier to cope with a very serious problem. The right medication can help a person onto the right track. When the feelings of deep depression lift, the other causes can be dealt with in a more positive way.

It is also possible to improve the production of neurotransmitters in the brain with exercise. It has been shown that regular exercise alters brain chemistry and improves your mood. It also improves the circulation and allows more oxygen to reach the brain. Vigorous aerobic exercise, such as running or brisk walking, encourages the production of natural morphine-like substances called *endorphins,* which have been linked to feelings of well-being.

Making your diet more healthy, and relaxing through aromatherapy, meditation, or reflexology, are other ways of restoring energy and the motivation to take charge of your life.

Simply talking to someone may help to improve your condition. Therapy is very helpful in many cases, with or without medication, depending on the person. As depression is often caused by incidents in your life that you may have pushed to the back of your mind, talking to a psychologist or other trained person could help you. Short-term therapy (twelve to twenty sessions) is used to concentrate on specific symptoms. It will help you to recognise and change negative thinking patterns that often contribute to depression. If you don't want to talk to a stranger, a close friend could be just as useful. Expressing your deepest thoughts, fears and worries can be the first step to recovery.

Reducing stress by taking time off, postponing some duties or cancelling appointments that are not essential are also part of the recovery process. Learn to say 'no' to demands that are not too important. Take a week off, or ask someone to help with tasks that seem too difficult to handle.

Negative thinking, such as self-criticism or a gloomy outlook, contribute greatly to a depressed mood; and it can become a habit that is hard to break. You could try to pull yourself up each time you have feelings of worthlessness or doom about the future. Recognise your negative thoughts as something you have to fight against, and they will stop taking control of your mood and dragging you down.

Try also to improve your relationship with others by not worrying too much about what they think of you, or thinking that you are responsible for them. Relax and be yourself.

When you emerge from depression you will feel relieved and strong. But it is important to be patient and to realise that healing can take time. Recovery can be uneven, like taking one step forward and two steps back. There are good days and bad. Enjoy the good days, and don't worry too much about the bad ones. You have already come a long way if you have recognised the problem and sought help. Keep going. You will recover fully and be able to look forward to feeling happy, confident, and proud.

Ten useful tips about depression

1. **Go to your doctor and ask for help.** Depression is an illness like any other, and the sooner you do something about it, the sooner you will start feeling better.

2. **Talk to someone**—a therapist or close friend. Talking through your feelings is a great help when you are feeling sad.

3. **Learn to recognise the signs of a low mood.** Try to stop thinking in a negative way. Pull yourself up and say: stop!

4. **Try not to be too hard on yourself.** If you are having a bad day, learn to accept it. Everyone has bad days.

5. **Take up exercise.** It will alter the chemicals in your brain and make you feel better instantly.

6. **Get involved in social activities**—a bridge club, book club, bingo, sewing circle, or something that involves sport. You may feel like avoiding other people, which is counterproductive when you are trying to combat depression.

7. **Be proud of every achievement**, even a small one. If you managed to go shopping, do some gardening, or go for a walk, reward yourself, even if you hated every moment.

8. **Remember that motivation comes after action.** Do things even if you don't feel like it: once you start you will want to keep going.

9. **Avoid alcohol.** You may feel it lifts your mood for a while, but alcohol is a depressant, which leaves you feeling even worse in the end.

10. **Reduce stress** by cutting down on commitments, by resting, and doing things you enjoy. Learning relaxation techniques through yoga and meditation is also helpful.

Useful addresses

Aware: Helping to Defeat Depression

147 Phibsborough Road

Dublin 7

Help line: (01) 6791711

Irish Hospice Foundation [bereavement support]

64 Waterloo Road

Dublin 4

Phone: (01) 6603111

Samaritans

112 Marlborough Street

Dublin 1

Phone: (01) 8727700

Help line: 1850 609090

In Britain

Depressive Self-Help Group

21 Morningside Gardens

Edinburgh E11 10SL

Scotland

Samaritans

PO box 9090

Slough, Berks SL1 1UU

Phone: (01345) 909090

The Depression Alliance [the leading self-help organisation for people with depression and their families]

Phone: (0171) 6339929

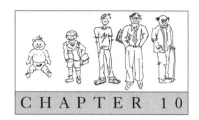

CHAPTER 10

THE TIME OF YOUR LIFE

LOOKING AFTER YOURSELF AND FEELING HAPPY

'Happiness is a butterfly which, when pursued, is always beyond our
grasp, but which, if you sit down quietly, may alight on you.'
—Nathaniel Hawthorne.

We all want to be happy. But ideas of happiness are individual; they also change with age. Happiness for a young person has often more to do with material things and being accepted by one's peers. Health, nature and peace of mind are things they take for granted and often don't even notice.

When I was a teenager I thought happiness was having no spots, getting into a size 10 skirt, and being asked to parties. Later, things that made me happy changed to being able to pay the mortgage, to the children going to sleep without a fight, to appreciating good health, love, family, friends, the beauty of nature, and above all, peace of mind.

Feeling well is very important to our mental health. It is difficult to feel happy if you are ill or in pain. Looking after your body by adopting a healthy life-style (as described in this book) will give you a feeling of well-being and help you enjoy the good things in life.

Older people often find it easier to be happy than younger people, strange as it may seem. When we are older we appreciate the simple things in life. We have time to contemplate the beauty of nature, we are more tolerant of other people, and we are grateful to feel well. Older people have more often than not been through hard times, which may have changed the way they look at life.

Our spiritual life is often richer when we are older. We may have found faith in God, or our faith may have become stronger. Some people may decide that they do not believe in God, and still have found a deeper meaning in life.

The smaller things in life make us feel happy and content. A delicious meal, a good laugh, a beautiful sunset, a chat with a friend or an enjoyable film are all things that bring joy into our lives.

W. M. Thackeray wrote: 'Respect your dinner, idolise it, enjoy it properly. You will be by many hours in the week, many weeks in the year, and many years in your life, the happier if you do.'

Abraham Lincoln is supposed to have said: 'Do not worry; eat three square meals a day; say your prayers; be courteous to your creditors; keep your digestion good; exercise, go slow and easy. Maybe there are other things your special case requires to make you happy, but my friend, these I reckon will give you a good lift.' Diet, exercise, faith in God, paying his debts and relaxing seem to have been Lincoln's recipe for happiness. It sounds easy, and to him, perhaps, it was.

Though we are born with a certain amount of optimism or pessimism, we can improve the way we feel about life. Studies on twins showed that about 46 per cent of personality is genetic. That is why some people seem naturally happier than others, even if they have to face hard times. Identical twins are likely to feel the same level of happiness, even if they have been separated at birth and have had a completely different upbringing.

The other half of our personality is up to ourselves. It is possible to change from being a pessimist to someone with a more positive outlook, though some of us may have to work a little harder to overcome a glum way of looking at things.

Living in the present

Living in the present is the most important way to feel happy. Living now, and not expecting to feel better in the future, is the key to happiness. You find happiness in your inner self, not somewhere out there in the future.

People are often unhappy because of fears and worries about what may happen in the future. We can spend all week worrying about a difficult decision or things that might happen to us.

You have to live in the moment. When you are watching a film, reading a book, or listening to music, do just that: don't think about other things. When you are gardening, garden. Live for now, and don't worry about things that are going to happen in a few hours' time.

That's not to say that you must not make plans. Of course you should. But don't expect things to be better or worse in the future. There is only now!

Pursuing happiness

You may also become addicted to the pursuit of happiness. You work hard to realise a dream, thinking that the result will make you happy. But it is the pursuit that becomes the goal, rather than the result. You are not prepared for the happiness when it arrives. You miss the chase, and the result is highly disappointing. For example, you may have worked and saved to buy a new car, go on an expensive holiday, or buy a bigger house. When the hard work has come to an end and you have the thing you have worked so hard for, you may discover that it was the hard work and the dream you enjoyed, not the achievement. In other words, the journey was more important than the arrival. If you accept that it is the journey that is the best part of the dream, you will enjoy life more.

It is important to take time to put your life into perspective. Deciding the direction you want to take makes you feel more in control. The more in control you feel, the happier you are.

Feeling happy makes us healthy

Simple pleasures, such as daydreaming or the smell of our favourite food, not only make us feel good but boost our health. The result of recent research showed that exposure to the smell of food such as chocolate, or remembering a happy event, produced an increase in the immune-boosting antibody SigA. The immune response lasted several days and seemed to give protection against respiratory infections. This proves that there is a direct link between moods and the immune system. In other words, feeling happy makes you healthy.

Another study showed that keeping secrets about painful or embarrassing experiences can lead to aches, colds, and fatigue; talking about it reduced the symptoms in 90 per cent of the subjects. (One wonders how some of these studies are done!) This could also explain why stress is so bad for us, and why even lack of sleep and feeling down can damage our health.

Stress

'Stress' is a modern concept. The term is used to describe a wide variety of emotions, such as worry, panic, nervousness, tension, or unhappiness. Stress can have a negative effect on our health by causing headaches and other pains and tension in our muscles. It can also increase blood pressure.

Stress is not all bad, however. A certain amount of it is good for us: it motivates us to try harder, to meet challenges, and to perform difficult tasks. Without some stress we would not be able to cope with moving house, meeting deadlines, getting through exams, or even doing the weekly shopping.

It can be pleasurable to feel stressed; but then we call it excitement. Certain sports with an element of danger or competition are hugely enjoyable to some people. When the danger is over there is a great feeling of pleasure. We are happy to have met a challenge and to have overcome it, or to have faced danger and survived.

 ## What can cause stress?

Stress can be emotional, physical, or environmental.

Emotional stress can be caused by a number of things: the death of a spouse or close relative, divorce, serious illness, moving house, retirement, problems at work, difficult relationships, money worries, taking tests, going for job interviews, and many more.

Physical stress, while not as serious, is also detrimental to our health. It is usually caused by injury, strenuous physical labour (such as carrying heavy objects), and over-exercising.

Environmental stress has to do with the air we breathe, noise levels, and the temperature we are exposed to.

All types of stress cause both mental and physical symptoms, some of them serious enough to damage health.

 ## What stress does to our bodies

When we are faced with a stressful situation, the body responds by preparing us for 'fight or flight' (as mentioned in chapter 5). We are programmed to either fight the danger or run away.

Emotions such as anger or fear trigger the release of the stress hormones *adrenaline, noradrenaline,* and *cortisol.* These in turn cause certain nerve responses in the body: the production of saliva decreases, and the mouth feels dry; the heart beats faster, and blood pressure increases; we start to sweat and to breathe faster, and the muscles contract, ready for action. Even the bladder and bowel can be affected: we can get diarrhoea and feel an urgent need to urinate.

All these responses, along with other complex ones, take place in an instant. When the danger has passed and we have dealt with it in one way or another, the stress hormones are no longer present. We feel exhausted. It is then important to relax.

These physical changes were useful for Stone Age people, who had no problem dealing with such an emergency: they either fought or ran away. It is more complicated for modern people. We don't respond only to danger: these reactions can be caused by facing a difficult task, rushing to catch a bus, dealing with problems at work, or arguing with colleagues. We often don't allow ourselves time to relax after having gone through a stressful situation but keep pushing ourselves to handle more stress. The body is forced to cope with more and more pressure, until it breaks down in some way.

How we cope with stress is very individual. Some people are introverted and pessimistic; they are most prone to chronic stress, such as loneliness. Even extroverts and highly organised people are likely to suffer from stress, because they don't take time to relax and to recover from the hectic pace of their lives.

Then there are the 'type A' and 'type B' personalities, so popular in the press. Type A is supposed to be aggressive and impatient, type B calm, slow, and patient. Some of us may lean towards the type A characteristics, others to type B, but we are probably all a mixture of A and B.

As we grow older we often have to face hardships such as bereavement, loneliness, and illness. Retirement and worry about money can also cause stress. We may have to care for older relatives, and help our children either financially or by taking care of grandchildren. While it is true that being needed and useful is positive, it is important to take time for ourselves from time to time.

How to relax

As stress-related illnesses and conditions are caused more by the lack of relaxation than stress itself, learning to relax is important. We need to relax both physically and mentally. By taking time to rest we are able to release accumulated mental and physical tension and restore energy levels.

Physical relaxation includes both exercise and rest. Exercise releases built-up tension and makes your body strong and fit; it also provides a complete break from everyday problems and concerns. Your blood circulation improves, and the feeling of well-being improves your mood. Resting allows the body to slow down and restore some of its lost energy. It is also good for the mind. There should be an equal balance between exercise and relaxation.

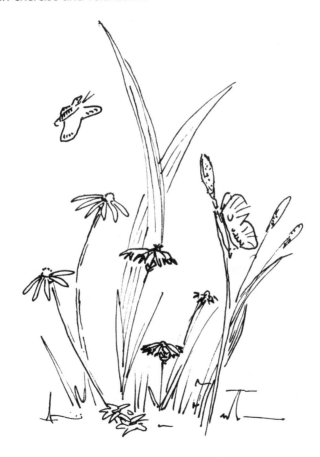

In chapter 4 we saw how to exercise and how to adopt a good exercise routine. There are many ways to keep physically active. Find something that suits you and that you enjoy. Regular exercise is a great way to beat stress.

Taking time off just to relax may seem self-indulgent to people who have a lot of commitments. Relaxing is not just sleeping or resting. You can relax by reading, listening to music, or watching television. Taking up activities such as yoga or stretching, having a massage or learning breathing techniques can be very soothing and comforting. The important thing is to slow down, take time to think, and have a little space just for you.

A good night's sleep

Sleep is important because it gives the body a chance to recover from the day's activities and allows the brain to process all the information it has received during the day. While we sleep, the endocrine system releases growth hormones, which repair and regenerate tissues.

Insomnia is a common problem among older people. It is generally believed that the older we get, the less sleep we need; you sometimes hear that very old people need only about four hours' sleep a night. This is not true. We need about eight hours' sleep a night all through life, though some people, for no apparent reason, seem to be able to manage on less.

The body clock that regulates sleep works just as efficiently when we are older. The reason older people have trouble sleeping is that they sleep more lightly, and their sleep gets gradually less and less deep. Because our sleep becomes less deep as we age, we are more likely to wake up early, and also to fall asleep during the day. While taking a short nap of about fifteen minutes is a good way to restore energy, sleeping for a longer period will disturb your nightly sleep pattern and make you wake up early. The best thing for coping with this may be to accept it, get used to waking up early, and enjoy your afternoon nap.

Another reason for poor sleep among older people may be nervousness about living alone, aches and pains, or other discomforts. In any case, anyone with severe insomnia should consult their doctor.

Results of studies show that exposure to light is a more important factor than previously believed in disrupting sleep. The tendency of many sleepless people to push bedtime later and later, particularly at weekends, has been blamed in some cases of sleeplessness.

If you are having trouble sleeping, try some of the following:

~ Have a cup of warm milk before going to bed. Milk contains an amino acid, *tryptophan,* that encourages the release of the sleep hormone.

~ Don't use alcohol as a way to make you sleep. Though alcohol makes you feel sleepy, it does not give you a good night's sleep. You may fall asleep quickly, only to wake up again and not be able to go back to sleep.

~ Read something soothing: poetry, a short story, or a novel. Don't read thrillers or stories that are so exciting you don't want to stop reading.

~ Have a warm bath (not too hot).

~ Go to bed at about the same time every night, and try to wake up at the same time.

~ Sleep in complete darkness.

~ Make sure your bedroom is neither too hot nor too cold and that there is enough ventilation (by keeping a window slightly open).

~ If your feet are cold, wear bed socks.

~ Open your curtains as soon as you wake up.

~ Make sure your mattress is not too hard or too soft and that your pillow supports your head without giving you a pain in the neck.

~ Don't worry about the occasional sleepless night. Try to relax, read something light, and remember that even if your mind feels alert, your body is resting.

~ Try to forget your worries. Put off solving problems until the next day: you can't do anything about them while you are in bed anyway.

Though it is important to get the right amount of sleep, too much rest is not good. Even when we are ill we shouldn't stay in bed too readily. A recent article in the *Lancet* (a British medical journal) revealed that bed rest is not good as a remedy for most illnesses. Of course people who are very weak as a result of an illness have little choice but to stay in bed; but the latest research suggests that even after medical procedures such as a lumbar puncture, spinal anaesthesia or cardiac catheterisation, the condition of patients worsened after bed rest. In patients suffering from acute low-back pain, high blood pressure, acute infectious hepatitis, or after labour or a heart attack, the result was the same. So we must try to keep going, even when we don't feel so well!

Self-image

As we grow older, we still want to look well—not only healthy, but attractive. Grooming is also pleasant and makes us feel good. Manicure, pedicure and regular visits to the dentist, hairdresser or barber make us both look and feel well. This is as important for men as for women. It is important to take pride in our appearance when we age. Women are probably better than men at looking after the way they look; older men have a tendency not to care much whether they look well or not.

We should take a little time each day to pamper our body. A daily shower or bath, followed by the application of body lotion, makes us feel well, both men and women. It helps soothe older, dry skin.

Foot care is important for health reasons. A once-weekly pedicure will keep your feet soft and comfortable and prevent problems. A good home pedicure is lovely and relaxing. Soak your feet in hot water for about fifteen minutes; scrub them with a pumice stone to remove dry skin; dry them vigorously with a towel, trim the nails, and rub in some foot lotion.

Regular visits to a chiropodist are also a good idea. Some older people have serious problems, such as athlete's foot, verrucas, bunions, corns, calluses, or chilblains.

Symptoms of athlete's foot (a fungal infection) are itching between the toes, flaking, and moist, broken skin. Over-the-counter remedies are effective, but the condition may take a few months to clear up. Change your shoes each day, and make sure your feet are completely dry before putting on tights or socks. You could also apply a little surgical spirit between each toe before getting dressed.

Verrucas are a form of wart caused by a viral infection, usually picked up in a damp environment, such as swimming-pools and communal showers. They can be very painful when standing or walking, and should be professionally treated by your GP.

Bunions (enlargements of the joint of the big toe) can be either genetic or caused by wearing tight shoes. They can be surgically removed, which is well worth the trouble if it causes serious pain.

Corns are caused by repeated chafing of badly fitted shoes. Do not try to cut corns yourself. Wear corn plasters from the chemist, or have them treated professionally.

Calluses—thickened skin, usually on the heels—can be removed with a pumice stone, or by the chiropodist.

Chilblains appear when the peripheral blood vessels in the feet are repeatedly constricted by warming the feet too quickly. The skin becomes red and itchy and then forms painful cracks. They can be soothed with calamine lotion. Keeping your feet warm by wearing good shoes in winter also helps

Look after your hands by massaging them with hand lotion every day. (Yes, men too!) This will keep skin soft and hands supple. Keep your nails trimmed.

Visit your dentist every six months, and take good care of your teeth by brushing and flossing every day. Keep your hair neat and tidy. Long hair does not look good on older men or women.

A little daily grooming is good for you and makes you feel fresh and clean.

Pet therapy

Animals can give us great pleasure. Medical research shows that keeping a pet can calm nervous disorders, ease loneliness, and speed up recovery from some illnesses. Stroking an animal reduces blood pressure. Walking your dog makes that daily walk more fun: it gives you a reason to go out and walk, as dogs need to be exercised every day. It can also help you meet other dog-owners, and thus make friends.

Keeping a dog is a continuous responsibility and a good way to feel that someone needs you. Dogs are particularly good at returning their owner's love. Cats also make lovely pets.

 Coping with retirement

Retirement completely changes your life. It can make you feel bored, lonely, and isolated. You may feel a lack of purpose, start worrying about money, and lose confidence.

You should plan both your financial situation and your activities a few years before the date of your retirement. A good way to prepare is to gradually cut back on your working hours, so that the change from your working life is not too sudden. Think of taking a part-time job or doing voluntary work when you retire, so that you will have something worthwhile to do. You will also meet people.

Plan your day as if you were going to work; organise time for shopping, gardening, housework, and walking. Make sure you meet people and do something you enjoy every day. Take up that hobby.

 Living alone

Loneliness is a problem that affects many older people. We may have to face living on our own at some stage in our life, usually when our partner dies and the children are long gone. Some people will have lived on their own all their adult life but find it more difficult to cope as they age. As we grow older we may find that many of our contemporaries have died and there are fewer people of our age group around.

Loneliness is not something we like to admit to, and many people keep their feelings to themselves; we don't want to lean on other people. But there is a lot we can do ourselves to feel less lonely.

Most people see only a small group of friends or family regularly. You may see members of your family only a few times a year, and your friends have perhaps died or moved away. Perhaps you have got into the habit of not seeing anyone for long periods. It is important to make a conscious effort to get out and see people. The best way to make friends is to join a club, take up a sport, or make yourself useful in your community. There are clubs, classes and sports activities in most communities. Ask at your local library, or study the notice board at the post office or the supermarket.

There may be other people just as lonely as you. If you are reasonably healthy, find out if someone near you needs help with shopping or housework, or just reading the newspaper. If you like small children there may be a young mother in the area who would be delighted with a little baby-sitting.

Don't forget your body language! If you look sad and grumpy, you will frighten people away. Try to look cheerful and positive. Remember how you feel yourself if someone smiles and seems happy. It's contagious, and you can't help liking that person. You may feel you have nothing to smile about, but you also have nothing to lose!

Having fun

Sadness and loneliness can rob you of your sense of fun. But laughing is good for us. It even improves our physical health: it increases the respiration, lowers blood pressure, exercises the heart muscle and internal organs, and builds up the immune system. Laughter lowers the level of the stress hormones and increases the number of white blood cells (which fight infection). If you find it difficult to laugh at anything in your daily life, rent a video or read a funny book. Or try to spend time with your funniest, most cheerful friends. Laughing about some of the difficulties in your life makes you feel more cheerful. As Mark Twain said, 'humour is the great thing, the saving thing after all; the minute it crops up, all our hardnesses yield, all our irritations and resentments flit away, and a sunny spirit takes their place.'

A final word

It's not easy to grow old. But life itself is not easy. Just as it is possible to feel unhappy at any age, it is also possible to feel happy and fulfilled all through life. Old people are generally content with their lives and cope very well with minor discomforts.

Being older brings with it many advantages. You feel calmer and more confident. You don't have to put up with the same stress and pressures as younger people. (If being young means having to juggle work, child care, and housework, I would rather be old!) You can be useful to your children and younger relatives by giving them help, advice, and comfort.

As an older person, you are part of a fast-growing population group. At the beginning of the twentieth century, one in twenty-five Europeans was aged sixty or over; by the year 2020, one in four people will be over sixty. Let's hope that the majority of us will be in good health.

Old people are more busy and involved in their communities than ever before. Retirement was formerly seen as the end of an active life; nowadays it is seen as a chance to do something different. More and more retired people take up activities and learn new skills. The elderly are becoming increasingly fit and active.

If you follow the advice in this book and look after your health by taking exercise, eating a healthy diet, and having regular medical check-ups, you will have a good quality of life, whatever your age. If you feel well and strong you will enjoy life more. As motivation comes after action, don't wait to feel motivated to start. Do it now!

Being older does not mean the beginning of the end of an active life: it is the chance to start something new. If you are already fit and well and used to regular exercise, keep it up! If you have not been very active before, remember, it's never too late to start. Look after yourself. Enjoy the age you are, and make the best of it.

Time is—the present moment well employ.
Time was—is past—thou canst not it enjoy.
Time future—is not and may never be.
Time present is the only time for thee.
                              —Anonymous (eighteenth century).

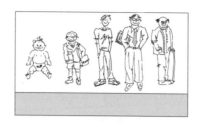

HELPFUL
ORGANISATIONS

Age Action Ireland

30 Lower Camden Street

Dublin 2

Phone: (01) 4756989

A national non-governmental organisation covering a network of associations that provide services for older people, including information, a library, a monthly bulletin, and a directory of services for older people.

Federation of Active Retirement Associations

59 Dame Street

Dublin 2

Phone: (01) 6792142

An umbrella body for the network of active retirement associations around Ireland, run for and by local retired people, who organise many activities for members.

National Council on Ageing and Older People

22 Clanwilliam Square

Dublin 2

Phone: (01) 6766484

An advisory body to the Minister for Health and Children on all aspects of ageing and the welfare of older people. It researches issues of particular interest to policy-makers. A list of publications is available from the council.

Retirement Planning Council of Ireland

27–29 Lower Pembroke Street

Dublin 2

Phone: (01) 6613139

Offers a free counselling service on all retirement matters and organises retirement preparation courses for companies and individuals.

In Britain

Age Concern

Phone: (020) 87657200

Fax: (020) 87657211

Web site: ageconcern.co.uk

In its role as the National Council on Ageing, Age Concern brings together the network of 1,400 local Age Concern organisations and over a hundred national organisations (including the main professional bodies and pensioners' organisations), which makes it the leading charitable movement in Britain concerned with ageing and older people. Local organisations provide vital services for older people in their areas, including day centres, lunch clubs, home visits, and transport services.